AIDS INC.

Scandal
of the
Century

by Jon Rappoport

First Edition

HUMAN ENERGY PRESS
Suite 205
1020 Foster City Boulevard
Foster City, California 94404

This book is a critical review of the scientific and social responses to AIDS. As such, it makes no recommendations about medical care, and no statement herein should be taken as medical advice. If people reading this book, or hearing about it, make decisions about their health or medical care which they believe are based on ideas contained in **AIDS INC.**, that is their constitutional right; the author and publisher assume no responsibility for such decisions or their implications.

Library of Congress: 88-080560
ISBN: 0-941523-03-9

Printed in the United States of America

CONTENTS

AUTHOR'S NOTE

No person I interviewed in writing this book necessarily ascribes to its conclusions.

I found many researchers making separate trains, took their snapshots, which I then arranged in my own way.

Many thanks, for specific research assistance, to Carla Valentine, Deborah Widel, Stace Aspey, Robin Babou, and Cheri Woods.

Thanks to Tamma Adamek for typing drafts of the manuscript and for assisting in the design of the book.

There are a hundred or so other people who contributed information, helped decipher journal articles, commented on AIDS research at the federal level, provided names and leads. My thanks to all of them.

Many books on scientific subjects illustrate their points with animal-experiments. It doesn't take long to realize, reading medical literature, that you can often take the animal research which agrees with your own conclusions and then just throw out the equally large stack of dissenting opinion. In fact, that is what some AIDS researchers do. So when I mention specific animal research in this book, I do so for one reason: to illustrate that very process, in which experiments that don't prove the party line are elbowed into oblivion.

There are several researchers who state that questioning the HIV virus as the cause of AIDS amounts to advocating promiscuity, free-for-all sex, and death for millions. This is absurd. The fact is, traditional sexually transmitted diseases, and the massive antibiotic-dosing that goes with repeated incidents of these diseases, is very immunosuppressive. So one doesn't have to swear allegiance to current AIDS research to favor safer sex.

I went back to my doctor and told him that I was better. Tests showed my T-cell count was improving. I had more energy.

He said I probably had AIDS dementia, and that's why I imagined I was getting well.

An AIDS patient, Los Angeles, 1988

The following is a brief exchange between a law professor and a physician. It concerns a volunteer subject in an experimental drug study of behavioral control, being conducted at a Maryland prison.

Law Professor: Does he (the volunteer) understand the effects of the drug?

Physician: Yes, we explained the whole thing to him. We don't want any misunderstanding.

Law Professor: Well, what are the effects?

Physician: We don't know. That's what we're trying to find out.

Recounted in Kind and Usual Punishment, *by Jessica Mitford (Alfred A Knopf, 1974).*

FOREWORD

Science-media myths shattered; Hope revealed! **AIDS INC.** is a powerful statement about the true cause of AIDS. The "cure" follows naturally.

Jon Rappoport has studied the scientific, political, and media responses to AIDS, and he provides an explanation which differs from what you have heard heretofore. A virus model of causation does not fit the scientific facts. Rather, multifactorial influences are the *sine qua non* of AIDS. The multifactorial model is a threat to the well-being of the international pharmaceutical giants, megalithic national research institutions, and aspirant Nobel Laureates. Most devastatingly, this model does not extrapolate to a single magic bullet cure. Rappoport suggests that we are headed in the wrong direction both socially and scientifically. Like the cancer epidemic, the AIDS epidemic is a harbinger of future disaster.

The story that Rappoport tells is not pleasant, and initially it will not be popular. From the ivory towers of science it is sure to be proclaimed "a heresy" and "an aberration." But, Rappoport has done his homework. Through countless hours of sleuthing about the libraries and halls of science, he has discovered the Achilles heels of the scientists and their theories. He has told his story with enough authority for it to be heard within these very halls of science. Truth is sometimes neither popular nor pretty. In **AIDS INC.**, human greed for money and power is revealed. An "old boys" network abounds within our federally regulated research institutions, and our leaders bear the shame.

The concept that AIDS represents the confluence of many different factors within the "modern" lifestyle is easy to understand. That a disease syndrome emerges in the latter part of the twentieth century as the result of historically unprecedented sexual promiscuity, drug abuse, promiscuous use of pharmaceuticals, rampant sexually transmitted diseases, widespread malnutrition (even in the U.S., where processed foods are common), and massive vaccination campaigns is plausible. The multifactorial explanation is further buttressed by the evidence that AIDS is occurring in those subsets of the population which participate in these injurious negative co-factors. Finally, the death knell of the virus-causation theory of AIDS is heralded by the identification of a few different viruses related to the cause. Never has there been one disease caused by different germs.

Truth is usually simple. Yet the AIDS virus theory has entered a realm of scientific obfuscation. Our addiction to animal research provides us with faulty information about AIDS and drugs intended for humans, who differ physiologically from other species. In the entire world today there are only approximately 200 scientists who understand the inner-circle language and symbols of esoteric virology. From sterile and isolated sancta, these "Priests of Virology" have handed down their own interpretations of the "Higher Knowledge" of Nature. These few Priests have informed the millions of doctors of the world as to "how things are" with this disease called AIDS. They have dazzled us with their exotic symbols and the relinquary tools of their "Laboratories!" They have blinded us to the nourishing environments we are immersed in daily. Yet it is precisely the breakdown in the dynamic balance of our sustaining environments which causes primary immune system weakness. Critical mass has been reached for AIDS. Rappoport has chronicled these events.

By the time you have finished **AIDS INC.**, you will understand why the AIDS virus is a relatively non-virulent opportunistic interloper, which takes advantage of a man-made situation. You will learn the true nature of immune system insults which afflict us all. You will understand why the AIDS epidemic, and other epidemics which are sure to follow, will not abate until man changes his situation. You will learn the truth, you will change your mind, and you will set yourself free.

Laurence E. Badgley, M.D.
July, 1988

AIDS INC.

INTRODUCTION

In the course of writing this book, I found many scientists who wouldn't talk on the record. They felt their jobs or grant monies would be jeopardized if they backed up their grievances–and they had serious grievances about the way AIDS is being researched and explained to Americans.

Is the machinery in place to stop "the plague" called AIDS? I believe, confirming these scientists' worst fears, that every major assumption about this syndrome, this disease, is wrong or in serious trouble.

Among patients there are massive desertions in the ranks. People with AIDS are searching out their own remedies, organizing their own studies, and in doing it, they're by and large spending less money than they would on orthodox care.

Meanwhile, medical powers-that-be are redefining AIDS. One virus, HIV, is now being asked to explain a huge, discordant series of physical symptoms. Failure in this is a certainty. It is the most embarrassing example of second-rate science in decades.

Set one undergraduate biology major loose in a library for a week, and he would be able to uncover legitimate journal-evidence that AIDS has a clinical face different from the one painted by NIH (National Institutes of Health).

In other words, with a shift in personnel at the top of the research ladder, overnight we would observe a considerably different AIDS than the one we are now being presented. Science...not a simple matter of truth, but a personnel problem.

AIDS is not the first instance of this, but AIDS will probably become the most damaging scandal the American medical orthodoxy has yet seen–while people die.

The organization responsible for finding an AIDS cure, NIH, operates in certain respects like any large corporation. Its cast of characters is production-oriented, competitive. Top-flight players try to establish domination, cut divergent thinkers out of the budget. These players of course also advertise their own stories of success. If that

1

means talking half-truths, spreading glitz to cover a lack of substance–there are PR people to handle that.

The above paragraph was a basic assumption I made in the spring of 1987, when I started researching AIDS. I've never found reason to reject this picture.

These days, at NIH, and at the Centers for Disease Control (CDC), the glossy advertisments are beginning to peel. Leaders are adjusting their toupees in the mirror. Beyond the scope of their machinations, the charade is coming to a close.

Jon Rappoport
Los Angeles

PART ONE

THE UNPROVEN AIDS EPIDEMIC

CHAPTER ONE

AIDS ON TV

Face it, what most of us know about AIDS comes through our television sets. But because information on AIDS is scientific, it's hard to be selective. We aren't doctors. Therefore, we have to trust that what we are seeing and hearing is true.

Unfortunately, that is a mistake.

AIDS is a word which, through repetition, has become a sword, a piece of hypnotic death-dealing.

Suppose I sit you down in front of a TV set and show you pictures I've strung together of black Africans, all skin and bones, walking slowly, stiffly, along a dirt road. Holding hands. They all have the most tentative movements.

Slowly, at the bottom of the screen, I have large red letters begin to emerge: AIDS. The voiceover gives us something like this: "Now it's making people blind. The cruelest killer of all. Get information. Save your life."

Of course, it's river blindness, not AIDS. But you watch a fictional ad like this over the course of a month and what will you believe?

When you have death and dying to work with in picture-form, the PR people who can get a chilling message across are a dime a dozen. Any death can be linked with *any* reason.

But how about this?

A man stands against a black backdrop, holding a small bottle of liquid. "See this?" he says. "Isobutyl nitrite. I know, you've never heard of it. People call it poppers. I sniffed this four times a week for three years. I have AIDS. Under this shirt, I have lesions on my arms. The first 50 AIDS patients *all* sniffed this. Of course, it isn't illegal, except in New York, Wisconsin, and Massachusetts. Your fed-

5

eral government refuses to take action against poppers. You can buy them over the counter. I wouldn't advise it, though."

You aren't seeing *that* on TV.

Now, as most of us realize, the people who fashion ads and PR aren't paid to know about the quality of what they are promoting. Their skills and their jobs have to do with building convincing images, period.

Suppose, in the case of AIDS, we are being fed "knowledge" which, originally, is based on inaccurate science, which is coming from sources which have overlooked very significant facts about the hysteria we are calling AIDS.

In that case, we would have, by now, a truly massive amount of distortion going. We would have speculation parading as fact, and we would have omissions on a grand scale.

This is, in fact, what we have.

Unfortunately, as I'll cover in more detail later, the media are not analysts of science. Even writers for the major newspapers in America, though a few are doctors, take their information direct from the press representatives at major federal health agencies. These press people are hardworking and helpful folks, but they are merely fed information by supervisors who run labs where research is carried on. The press people make *no* judgments on the accuracy of what they pass on to reporters.

Just in case you didn't know.

So it really isn't hard to imagine that, if wrong information starts at the top of the waterfall, by the time it cascades out into your livingroom through the tube, it is a disaster. But by that point, it has the ring of casual authority the media know how to impart. That is their business.

Another example. You know those TV pictures that show the HIV virus, the purported AIDS virus, chewing up the T-cells of our immune systems? Well, most people believe that those pictures are photos, or at least computer simulations made, dot by dot, of something that has definitely occurred and been observed inside the body.

I asked an eminent molecular biologist if that was true. He said, "No. It's a *complete* simulation. I'm not saying the TV depiction is intentionally phony, but what they're showing you is an invention. In fact, there is no proof that HIV viruses are doing that to your cells."

I believe the truth about AIDS, once it is dug out, is better news than what you've been hearing. You'll have to be the judge of that after you read this book. But on the whole, behind the media glaze, behind the hysteria, behind labs and researchers who are wedded to their theories, beyond even the illness and the dying there is some relief.

I would summarize the media position on AIDS as follows:

1. It is contagious. The virus has spread over much of the known world.
2. AIDS is invariably fatal.
3. It may well become another grand plague.

I'm going to offer evidence that none of these positions is true.

CHAPTER TWO

DYING OF WHAT?

In a house on Vermont Avenue, in Los Angeles, a twenty-five-year-old man with a chalky face is dying of AIDS. He sits in a chair propped up by pillows, covered with a blanket, and watches television.

Outside, in the back yard, I talk with his parents. The husband, a short stocky man who has spent most of his life tending bar in Sacramento, tells me something is wrong.

Wrong? Everyone knows the son is dying. What could be wrong, outside of that?

The mother nods in agreement with her husband.

"I don't think this is AIDS," the father says. "They've diagnosed him, but this whole thing has to do with drugs he had in Vietnam."

I look at the wife. She says, "He was all right until he came home. I mean, before he went off to fight there was nothing wrong with him. After the war, he began losing weight. He was miserable. He came back for awhile, got himself a job, but then he began to fade again."

"What about the AIDS virus," I say. "He has it, doesn't he?"

His father looks at me. "This isn't viruses. It's one of those damn pesticides, or heroin."

The conviction in his voice is absolute, and he doesn't sound like a man trying to pretend his son isn't homosexual.

Besides, the conversation isn't the first time I've been through something strange like this.

There was a man in San Francisco who was dying, too. Wasting away. His sister, a teacher, was taking care of him. One night, after supper, she said to me, "I've talked to his doctor for over an hour, and I don't think this physician knows what AIDS is. He explains it, and it just doesn't make sense."

9

She drags out a number of articles from medical journals and shows me passages that are checked off. She builds a case for AIDS as a mistaken label for syphilis. Syphilis, the disease called the great pretender, which has shown up over the centuries in many guises. She then hands me a list of street drugs with an "adverse effects" column next to each one. The symptoms do remind me of AIDS.

Then, in Venice, California, there was a man who had just been diagnosed as having AIDS. He called me through a mutual friend, told me he wanted to give me information for the book I was writing.

"I have no symptoms," he said. "I just tested positive for the HIV virus and my doctor wants to give me the drug, AZT. He says I have AIDS."

This sounds preposterous.

I ask, "How can he diagnose AIDS with only a blood test? Are you feeling sick?"

"I feel fine!" the man says. "My doctor tells me because I had headaches recently, the AIDS virus is probably in my brain." He laughs. "It's insane."

That night, we meet for dinner. He tells me he knows three or four people whose doctors have started them on AZT, the AIDS treatment, just because they tested positive for the AIDS virus. No symptoms.

AZT is a highly toxic drug that damages bone marrow and causes anemia. People who take it become so anemic they often need blood replacement by transfusion. So why in the world should a person who has no symptoms be taking such a drug?

Several reporters in New York had already told me about people with no symptoms who tested positive on AIDS blood tests – they were also being given AZT.

Then there was a woman in San Diego I met. She had been diagnosed with AIDS. She was an IV drug user who had recently stopped dealing and using heroin.

In a ridiculous setting, riding the elevated rail through the huge San Diego Zoo, she turned to me and said, "Don't believe everything you read in the papers about AIDS."

"Did you share needles?" I asked her.

She shook her head. "I'm not stupid. Do doctors in hospitals shoot two or three patients with the same needle, without cleaning it? Forget this thing about the AIDS virus getting passed around on needles. What gets passed around is drugs. Why don't they find out what's in the drugs?"

"Such as?"

She looked at me. "Keep trying," she said. "You'll figure it out."

All of the above conversations took place in the spring of 1987, just as I was beginning this book.

In July, I met a physician who was seeing AIDS patients in New York. He was out in Los Angeles on vacation, and I was introduced to him at an AIDS conference.

He started asking me questions about my book, about the articles I'd just been publishing on possible origins of AIDS.

After lunch, in the lobby of the hotel where the conference was being held, he handed me a folder. It contained a computer printout.

"Check out the citations," he said. "It'll make a good start for your book." He didn't want to talk further. With a quick wave, he walked out the door.

In the parking lot, I opened up the folder and found the printout was a long list of journal citations for articles about AIDS blood-testing. As it turned out, a number of them referred to the unreliability of those tests.

I found studies on my own which also rejected the idea that the blood tests were useful.

At this point, I decided to retreat to orthodox information on AIDS. I read a number of pamphlets and brochures put out by the National Institutes of Health (NIH) and the Centers for Disease Control (CDC), the two health agencies responsible for much of the research and statistics-keeping on AIDS. From these info sheets, and from several conversations with middle-of-the road researchers, I assembled a sample dialogue, questions and answers on AIDS. Everything in black and white. It is meant to form the background for the discussion of AIDS in this book.

AIDS patients are dying, but of what?

Of infections and illnesses. Various kinds.

For instance?

Pneumocystis pneumonia.

What's new about that?

The reason these people come down with pneumocystis is new. The reason is a virus.

HIV?

Yes. Human immunodeficiency virus, the AIDS virus.

What does it do?

It damages the immune system, which would ordinarily respond to germs and destroy them.

So now the immune system can't defeat ordinary illness.

Now harmless or mild germs like pneumocystis become very dangerous, even lethal.

And that's AIDS.

Yes.

What part of the immune system does the HIV virus damage?

The T-cells. They are called T because they're manufactured in the thymus gland.

Is AIDS invariably fatal?

It seems so.

Is there a way to slow it down?

We have a drug to keep the HIV virus from spreading. It's called AZT.

Does HIV attack any other part of the immune system?

The macrophages. They are cells which are the first line of defense against illness. They move around the body eating up foreign germs.

HIV also attacks the spine and the brain. People who suffer from this brain infection often develop what's called AIDS dementia.

They actually act demented?

Eventually.

What is ARC?

12

AIDS-Related Complex. It's a pre-AIDS condition. The symptoms include night sweats, fever, diarrhea, swollen glands, and general malaise.

Do most people who get ARC then get AIDS?

Many do, yes. Perhaps 50%, perhaps more.

What are the symptoms of AIDS dementia?

The early symptoms are mental disorientation, forgetting names or appointments, perhaps leg weakness. This eventually becomes full-blown mental incompetence and confusion.

I've heard of a form of AIDS in Africa called slim disease.

Slim and AIDS are the same thing. In Africa and the Third World in general, one of the major symptoms of AIDS is severe weight-loss. Hence the name slim. The other major symptoms there are chronic diarrhea and chronic fever.

But it's still AIDS. The HIV virus is weakening the immune system, allowing the fever and weight-loss and diarrhea to occur and persist.

Yes.

In the United States, is slim part of AIDS?

Definitely. We call it the wasting syndrome. You lose weight, a considerable amount. Wasting is on the list of infections and diseases which are unmistakably bold signs of AIDS.

So slim, AIDS, pre-AIDS, these are all in one way or another part of the same disease-picture.

That's right.

If you test positive on an AIDS blood test, does that mean you have AIDS?

No. It means you have contacted, been exposed to the HIV virus. Some people call this being infected by HIV, which is technically incorrect. But later on, perhaps many years in the future, you may very well contract AIDS.

What are the exact symptoms of full-blown AIDS, the fatal disease?

Until recently, you had to test positive for the presence of HIV and you also had to have one or more infections or diseases from a list, which are called AIDS indicator diseases. The two most prevalent of these are pneumocystis carinii pneumonia and Kaposi's sarcoma, which is a cancer of the blood vessels.

But there are other AIDS indicator diseases?

Many. About thirty.

Do you still have to test positive for the HIV virus in order to be diagnosed as having AIDS?

Not necessarily. As of September, 1987, you can have one of the indicator diseases and be diagnosed with AIDS, even though you don't show a definite, positive test for the HIV virus.

Six months after I had put together this little AIDS dialogue, I was appearing regularly as a late-night guest on KPFK, LA's Pacifica FM radio station. Roy Tuckman, host of the *Something's Happening* show, was having me on for three and four hours at a crack, and the call-in response was very good.

Once the station used a brief two-minute comment of mine for the morning news, and a day later I got a call from a man who had heard that broadcast and wanted to tell me about AIDS in San Francisco, the gay bathhouse scene there, in the 1970s, and the drugs that went with it.

His point meshed with one I was already finding central to a discussion of AIDS: drugs, alone, adulterated, or in combinations, can cause symptoms we call AIDS. No virus necessary.

His information, and other info like it, eventually put the cap on my research. I was able to collect a response to the official position on AIDS.

It is:

• There is no disease-entity which ought to be called AIDS. AIDS is not one thing.

• The HIV virus has never been proved to cause any disease of any kind.

• The treatment for AIDS patients, AZT, can be dangerous.

• No conclusive proof exists that we have a contagious epidemic *caused by a virus.*

•The AIDS blood tests which have existed up to May, 1988, are unreliable. And, of course, they are testing for exposure to a virus which has not been proven the cause of any illness.

•Efforts to develop an AIDS vaccine, likewise, are aimed at preventing infection by HIV, which has not been proved to be harmful to anybody.

•The various definitions of AIDS, used to make diagnoses around the world, are useless and vague. They allow almost anyone to be pinned with the label, AIDS. They actually function to terrorize people. They also, by semantic juggling, promote vastly increased numbers of AIDS cases, which naturally leads to the wide marketing of highly profitable pharmaceuticals as treatments.

•Official symptoms of pre-AIDS, AIDS, dementia, slim – whatever title you use – can all be accounted for by the effects of medical and street-drugs, or by older forms of illness.

•There is no proof that one malady called AIDS exists.

•Many episodes of traditional sexually transmitted diseases, like gonorrhea and syphilis, along with massive amounts of antibiotics, can cause a great deal of immunosuppression. Rejecting HIV as the cause of disease therefore does not imply an endorsement of free-for-all sex.

•The label AIDS has a devastating psychological and emotional impact. On close inspection, it means almost nothing. The closest synonym to it is Human Immune Suppression, which of course has hundreds of causes.

Naturally, in coming to these positions about AIDS, I spoke with a number of scientists and physicians. Surprisingly, I found many who disagreed with the official scenario on AIDS.

There were also people whose conclusions went a long way in shaping my own thoughts. Several of the interviews I held with them are reprinted in later chapters.

What I'm going to do in this book is give evidence for the positions I've just stated. Make a new map, one I believe is overdue.

What is AIDS actually, when you strip away the terroristic label? As I say, it is *not one thing*. It is any form of severe immunosuppression, *from any source*, which then gives rise to opportunistic infections.

These infections are sometimes unusual, because the microorganisms that cause them are benign under ordinary circumstances. But with the immune response lowered, the microorganisms come to the fore and behave virulently. This is the pattern for all forms of immune suppression. It always has been. It is nothing new. First, reduced immune response. Then, infections.

In every spot on the globe where AIDS is said to occur, we find researchers have avoided a thorough study, a ground-level examination of ingrained immunosuppressive factors that already exist.

For example, in the US gay communities of Los Angeles, New York, and San Francisco, most attempts to understand the so-called bathhouse lifestyle have been half-hearted. They have failed to examine at close range the incredible parade of immunosuppressive drugs, both medical and street-type, which have paraded through that scene in historically unprecedented quantities and combinations.

In Africa, a whole different set of traditional, and more recent immunosuppressive factors have been at work, and one of the crimes of second-rate medical research there has been the failure to really comb areas of the Central African republics and learn what is going on.

As you will see, many of the symptoms of what is called AIDS are the symptoms of toxic reactions to chemicals, or of already known illnesses.

But people insist on believing that AIDS is everywhere one condition caused by one thing, a virus.

Meanwhile, the death-sentence, *You have AIDS*, has the impact of a Medieval priest preparing a lapsed believer for Hell. In all the hype about AIDS, the severe psychosomatic effect of that death sentence is underplayed.

We also have hysteria about the *possibility* of contracting an invariably fatal disease. This might be understandable if it had been proved, really proved, that, with AIDS, we have a single-source epidemic on our hands. But that is not the case. From reports, many, many people diagnosed with AIDS were *already* suffering from considerable immunosuppression which had nothing to do with a virus. It had to do with exposure to drugs, to already known diseases.

There are several types of "synthetic AIDS" among heavy IV drug users, and none of them would require a virus to cause severe immune damage. Everything debilitating could be caused by chemicals. One striking example, documented, involves a ten-year period between 1973 and 1983, during which PharmChem Laboratories, in Menlo Park, California, analyzed samples of street drugs from all over the world. Among their many findings was the discovery that a drug called MPPP, a synthetic substitute sold as heroin, contained a byproduct called MPTP.

MPTP can cause a virtual case of Parkinson's disease from one injection. In fact, in 1985, the Santa Clara Valley Medical Center, in San Jose, California, set up an MPTP/Parkinson's clinic, since they were seeing increasing numbers of people afflicted by this drug.[1]

I asked whether these patients have been known to lose weight. "Oh yes," a clinic spokesperson told me. "It can be very dramatic, up to forty or fifty pounds."[2] In AIDS literature, such weight-loss is called the wasting syndrome. By the present CDC definition of AIDS, it is sufficient grounds for a diagnosis of AIDS. Other symptoms of MPTP include muscle ache and fatigue, associated with Pre-AIDS.

It is clear that an ordinary examining physician would completely miss the fact that his IV drug-using patient was suffering weight-loss from a chemical. He would have to understand the substitution, first, of MPPP for street heroin, and then the adulteration of *that* with MPTP. Not easy knowledge to come by.

Why have we not heard much about MPTP and other chemicals?

The medical research-machine is geared to collect symptoms, put them under umbrellas, uncover causative germs, and find drugs to treat those germs. It is not geared to analyze deeply the *deleterious*

---

[1]Conservative estimates by PharmChem indicate that 500 people in Central California were exposed to MPTP.

[2]A *part* of the weight-loss is due to treatment for Parkinson's.

effects of drugs which, in many cases, are not so different from medical preparations. Which in some cases, *are* medical preparations.

Two summers ago in New York, I met a man who had just been diagnosed with AIDS. The list of drugs he had used in his life or had been prescribed was several pages long. He was terribly frightened, but not of the cumulative effect of these drugs on his health. He was afraid of a virus; of, to be more exact, the AIDS death sentence he had just been delivered.

He told me that, although he had just had one mild episode of pneumonia, he felt he had no chance to recover. The die had been cast. He knew the AIDS treatment, AZT, was very bad for his immune system, but he was going to take it anyway. "What else can I do?" he said.

Since the diagnosis of AIDS, he was having trouble sleeping. He was afraid to tell his friends that he was "terminal." "I'm as good as dead," he said. "Maybe I should think about a trip to Holland. Euthanasia is legal there."

A week after I saw the man, he wrote me a letter:

"I feel like an institutionalized case, even though I've only been in a hospital once in my life. I see myself ending up in one, or in some hospice where they're very nice to me and whisper to me about dying, trying to make it easy. I say 'institutionalized' because I've been taking drugs all my life. I buy them from dealers and my doctors give them to me. That's all I know. How else can I cure AIDS unless I take another drug? I've always relied on one kind of chemical or another."

Just in case anyone thinks I'm an anti-drug moralist, let me give you some idea, some *partial* idea, of the drugs this man had regularly taken over a ten year period.

Starting in 1972, he had begun to use poppers, which are inhalant nitrite compounds. Serious drugs. They are snorted as both an orgasm-enhancer and a muscle relaxant, and were widely used in the gay bathhouse scene starting in about 1972. One researcher told me the carcinogenic potential of these nitrites is a *million* times that of the nitrites in bacon. This man, for seven years, did huge doses of poppers on the average of three times a week. The levels at which he was taking the drug will never be replicated in scientific studies, in humans, because they are inhumanly unethical.

For two years, he was supplied with poppers by his physician, not for any condition he was suffering, but as a recreational "favor." Then he went to the adulterated street versions, which are even more toxic than the pharmaceutical-grade stuff his doctor was giving him.

Ordinarily, during a weekend at the bathhouse, he also did, in concert with poppers, massive amounts of MDA, which is a speed-type drug with a sensual component (a sexual stimulant). He did MDA two or three times a night on Fridays and Saturdays, and once or twice on Sundays.

He also, on an average weekend, steadily ingested quaaludes (which, in 1980, began to be contaminated with a compound called ortho-toluidine, a brain toxin); did four or five valium; ten to twenty lines of cocaine; acid; ten to fifteen joints of marijuana (occasionally laced with the dangerous pesticide, paraquat); antibiotics, just in case he ran across sexually transmitted bacteria; and a quart or two of scotch.

This regimen went on for almost nine years.

During the week, he used heroin, at a rate of about two grains a day. When heroin was in short supply, or he didn't feel safe about the possible contaminants in it, he chewed percodans like candy. He also used pharmaceutical grade amphetamines which he obtained from his doctor, and during four or five periods favored this drug over heroin or percodans, suffering subsequent speed burnouts, physical and emotional depletions of considerable magnitude.

Meanwhile, because of his large numbers of sexually transmitted diseases, he kept on steadily with antibiotics, whether or not at any given moment he had an infection. In other words, on prescription from his doctor, he was popping tetracycline against the possibility that he might get sick. The problems with this approach to medication are spelled out in a later chapter – but suffice it to say, you can throw off completely the balance of friendly and unfriendly bacteria in your body with such a regimen, and you can also create large numbers of antibiotic-resistant germs.

Because he often suffered from inflammatory infections, he was also prescribed corticosteroids, which in one study[3] has been found, in concert with other compounds, to be very immunosuppressive, leading in fact to pneumocystis pneumonia, the major symptom of AIDS (32,000 cases of pneumocustis since 1980).

Then, to build muscle, he took several steroids on and off for six years.

There is more, but you get the idea.

In early 1988, this man wrote me a letter in which he said, "You know, I do find it curious that although several doctors have spoken to me about my past drug use, none of them has seriously suggested it could be responsible for my AIDS, or whatever the hell this illness is I have."

In the same letter, the man remarked that he had been taken off the AIDS treatment, AZT, because he needed too many blood transfusions. Of course, blood transfusions also open up the possibility of getting any number of germs placed directly into your bloodstream, without first passing through the ordinary portals of the immune system.

As will be discussed later, AZT, in attacking the bone marrow, has a severe, negative effect on the very immune system the AIDS patient is having problems with.

About three months ago, I received another letter from this man. He said he had had another episode of pneumocystis pneumonia.

He now had two doctors, and one of them was suggesting he might want to consider going to Holland, where euthanasia was possible – although he still wasn't bedridden, and was working a half-time job.

A "specialist in death and dying" was counseling him. He was beginning to get annoyed with these ministrations, and wrote, "I may just go off and try to get healthy on my own. Ridiculous as this sounds, it is even more ridiculous that I didn't consider this much, much earlier. Maybe it's too late for me, but I'd like to find out. Ev-

---

[3] *Journal of Immunology*, vol. 133, 1984, p. 2502.

eryone here is so geared to fatalism about AIDS. It's a kind of massive hypnotism. The expectation is that I'm going to die, and pretty soon. The date, exact date, is the only piece in the puzzle that's missing. I'm being lulled by well-meaning people into a death dance. They want to make it non-painful for me, but they become irritated when I tell them I want to fight this thing. I'm really so pissed-off I can't even begin to tell you about it. Something inside me is screaming. An injustice is being done. I've participated in it, but now that we're down to the tough part, everybody wants me to give up. I feel like I'm just waking up to the consequences of what happened over these last ten years and I don't want to lie down . . ."

I approached a physician I knew in New York who was treating AIDS patients, the same man who had put information in my hands about AIDS testing. I set in front of him the list, only partially described here, of the drugs this man had taken during a ten-year period.

Then I included a list of his symptoms. First, the pre-AIDS ones: diarrhea, swollen glands, night sweats, intermittent fevers, depression. Next, I added the infections which had brought on a diagnosis of AIDS: pneumocystis pneumonia, oral candidiasis (a fungal infection), staph, various skin rashes and inflammatory problems.

I asked the doctor whether these symptoms could have been caused, in full, by this man's ingestion of drugs over ten years.

He said, "I'm not going to go on the record with this, but you can find out by looking carefully through ordinary drug reference-texts and talking with people who take these street-drugs. I see nothing this man has suffered which couldn't have been brought on by the drugs, plus his history of sexually transmitted diseases."

"In other words," I said, "no virus, no HIV virus was necessary."

The doctor stared at me and nodded yes, as if he didn't want even the sound of his voice to somehow implicate him in medical heresy.

CHAPTER THREE

CAN A PRISON EXPERIMENT CAUSE AIDS?

Ken has kept a journal since his doctor told him he had AIDS in 1983. After two bouts of pneumocystis carinii pneumonia, he left his doctor and began treating himself.

"Tell your readers I'm black," he said to me pointedly the first time we spoke, over a year ago, "and tell them the rate of AIDS among blacks is twice as high, per capita, as among whites."[1]

In 1983, Ken decided he would begin using herbs for his condition, and he would try to detoxify "the poisons in my system."

This led him into many avenues of alternative treatment, and, like a number of other people with AIDS I've spoken to, he has refused to accept a permanent protocol for treatment from any MD, even a holistic one. In fact, among the AIDS survivors I've met, this independence of mind and self-doctoring seem to be the one common denominator.

Ken, 27, was working "in show business" in Los Angeles, until, in 1984, he was too weak to continue. He began a course of acupuncture, experimented with herbs from the Southwestern US, and after six months, started a high-dose course of vitamin C. He has also taken the lecithin compound, AL 721 (not approved by the FDA). He'll take baths in which he adds a very diluted amount of hydrogen peroxide.

His journal is a record of what appears to be a comeback from illness. He now runs a mile a day, swims twice a week and plays golf. He no longer works in show business, but holds down another full-time job.

"I know these treatments I've dosed myself with sound crazy," he tells me, "but all I care is they work for me. I don't recommend them for anyone. I can't tell what'll benefit another person. But I do

---

[1]The same is true for Hispanics.

feel very strongly that whatever I was suffering from, it's gone, and that AIDS isn't fatal. Doesn't have to be."

One of the entries in Ken's journal interested me:

"Try to find one study of people who have tested positive for the HIV virus. People with no symptoms. Track them over a few years and see what happens if they change their habits."

The habits he meant were monumental drug-taking and having hundreds (or thousands) of sexual partners, thereby increasing tremendously the risk of exposure to traditional sexual diseases.

I have looked in the literature, and have found no major study like the one he envisions. It is surprising when you think about it, because:

a) AIDS is supposed to be a disease that causes severe immune-suppression;

b) so if people who are supposedly at risk for AIDS cut out, from their lives, immunosuppressive habits, it's reasonable to wonder whether they'll enjoy better health and avoid debilitating illness.

No mainstream study of any proportions has been done on this subject. Much of the doom and gloom about AIDS stems from a different sort of ongoing study at the San Francisco City Clinic, several years long at this point. The two groups of men who constitute the study-samples are very specialized. They either participated in the original Hepatitis B vaccine trials in San Fran sco in 1980; or they had been showing up for diagnosis and treatment of sexually transmitted diseases at clinics in San Francisco, in the late 1970s. This latter group stood a good chance of already being immune-compromised from their sexual infections and a great deal of antibiotic-taking.

Reading through Ken's journal, I put together an interesting history of his drug-use. Interesting because it was relatively minor. A modest amount of cocaine in the late 1960s, pain pills for a bad back during the same period. Social booze.

But I found this cryptic reference: "Year and a half, facility treatment." No date, no name. I asked him about it. He had been generous in opening up his journal to me, saying he didn't really care about his past anymore, and that I could read through it. On the point of his incarceration, though, he was evasive.

Finally, he said, "Look, I was in a joint, and in this place they did experiments. On some of the inmates. Does that tell you something?"

He would say no more. But then a week or so later, he gave a stack of articles and books to take home with me. One was Jessica Mitford's *Kind and Usual Punishmemt* (Alfred A. Knopf, 1974), a well-known analysis of aspects of prison life in the US, including medical experimentation.

In the stack were also articles from several gay papers. One article was entitled "Atascadero–Dachau for Queers?"[2]

The October 9, 1970, issue of *Medical World News* made public what some people have known for decades. Those people who are classed as sexual deviants have been experimented on in mental facilities in the United States.

This article, *"Scaring the Devil Out,"* describes the use of a drug called succinylcholine at Atascadero state hospital for the criminally insane, in California, and at the California Medical Facility at Vacaville. The article notes that the drug has been used on some patients without informed consent, who have not been violent, who have engaged as inmates in "deviant sexual behavior," or who have been unresponsive to the hospital's group therapy programs:

"More than 100 men...have received 20 mg. to 40 mg. of succinylcholine. This dosage...is sufficient to induce general paralysis and respiratory arrest lasting up to two minutes."

While in a state of terror, feeling they might die, these patients would be lectured to by prison doctors, who would tell them that their behavior had to change.

Arthur Nugent, chief psychiatrist at Vacaville, told the *Medical World News:* "The prison grapevine works fast, and even the toughest have come to fear and hate the drug. I don't blame them. I wouldn't have the treatment myself for the world."

These and other "experiments" were later mentioned by John Lastala in his *Advocate* article, "Atascadero–Dachau for Queers?" Based on an interview with an unnamed inmate, Lastala cryptically

---

2 *The Advocate*, April 26, 1972

indicates that, "under threat of lifetime incarceration, sex offenders are being coerced into giving their consent for operations which leave them of little real value to anyone, least of all themselves."

Lastala cites the case of a 24-year-old homosexual prisoner at Vacaville who, after various experiments presumably done in conjunction with drug companies, went into a suicidal depression and was in serious physical condition "with ulcerated legs."

According to Lastala's informant, a drug called prolixin had replaced succinylcholine at Vacaville. This drug was sometimes administered in Ward 14, where inmates were transferred if they were caught in a homosexual act. There, the story goes, they were beaten, their heads were shaved, and they were put in walking restraints. They were kept there for from 3-6 months.

The inmate told Lastala that prolixin also induces extreme difficulty in breathing, and brings on a kind of psychedelic experience in which concentrating on a thought is impossible. "The doctors *tell* you you're dying...You're like a vegetable. You sweat. They tell you if you're ever caught having sex in here again you won't get the antidote."

It's estimated that about 8% of the inmates at Atascadero had been given this sort of drug, prior to 1972.

The inmate also stated that a process called "Errorless Extinction of Penile Responses" was practiced. Wires were attached to the inmate's penis. He sat in front of a screen and sexual pictures were flashed on it. If he got an erection, he was given electric shocks.

This practice was confirmed in 1970, when William Chambliss, a sociologist at the University of California, Santa Barbara, visited Atascadero, as part of a three-person committee empowered by the state's Department of Mental Health to look into the working of the institution.

Chambliss, after his visit, wrote, "I do not know what its patients and staff are like when they are not in the institution, but judging from their behavior there, I would feel a great deal more secure about the world if the patients went home at night and the staff stayed locked up."

I spoke with Chambliss recently, and he described a few of his experiences while at the facility.

"First of all," he said, "there are both violent offenders and people who are there because of incidents like voyeurism and exhibitionism. I saw perhaps 50 patients sitting around like zombies, from drugs which were used to make people change their behavior.

"The head psychologist told me, punctuating his remarks with little snickers and chuckles, 'We have this program of aversive therapy. We take these people–well, they volunteer, but they do because they want to get out–we attach their penises to wires and show them pictures of their deviation. If they become erect, we shock them until they don't become erect anymore.'"

Chambliss added, "We wrote up a very condemnatory report, and several people at Atascadero were fired. But we shouldn't imagine that that puts an end to this sort of thing, or to similar practices in other facilities. These practices are institutionalized. They're part of a system...they can find new people to continue them."

Jessica Mitford points out in *Kind and Usual Punishment* that, in 1962, a law suit was brought over a drug experiment conducted at Vacaville. The plaintiff had been a subject in pain-tolerance studies; a drug called Varidase was used. He developed a near-fatal muscular disease. His weight went from 140 to 75 pounds. Nineteen other subjects in this study suffered chills, sweating, sharp abdominal pains, exhaustion, rapid weight loss, headache, weakness.

Needless to say, these are now called AIDS and Pre-AIDS symptoms. It isn't easy to learn about the bulk of prison and military experiments which take place in this country, but one has to wonder when presented with a list of symptoms like these.

It is known that organophosphate pesticides have also been tested in the California prison system. Mitford points this out. Weight-loss, the so-called AIDS wasting syndrome, can occur from exposure to those chemicals as well. In other prison experiments, cardiac failure, finger-loss from decreased blood circulation, fungus infections, and neurological damage have resulted.

In 1973, according to Mitford, NIH funded a study at the Maryland House of Correction, in which cholera, typhoid, viral respiratory and viral diarrhea agents were injected in prisoners.

Ken asked me whether I enjoyed reading his literature on prison medical-experiments.

"What drugs did they give you?" I said.

"Don't you want to know why I was in a facility?" he asked. "It wasn't a violent crime. That's all you'll get to know...they gave me a drug—I'm not going to say the name. But I lost thirty-five pounds. Some days I thought I was going a little crazy. I got sick."

"You had infections?"

"Some funguses. They took a long time to go away."

I said, "I'm sure you know—today those fungus infections are on the list of AIDS diseases. So is the wasting away. Even forgetting the pneumocystis pneumonia, you could have been diagnosed with AIDS."

A week or so after this talk, I spoke with my anonymous doctor-friend in New York. I told him about Ken's symptoms.

"They might have given him Varidase," the doctor confirmed. "That could've given him those symptoms. Or large exposure to organophosphate pesticides could have been the experiment."

At this point, it became clearer to me that what people were calling AIDS could not only be produced by chemicals, without the need of a virus, but that the fundamental pattern of so-called AIDS—immune-suppression followed by various infections—could stem from a *variety of causes*.

When I told my physician friend this, he said, "That's blasphemy. People don't like that idea."

"Why not?"

"Well, first of all, they want HIV to be the thing that causes *all* immune-suppression in everyone. They want AIDS to be one horror story."

From my subsequent experience in talking to scientists and doctors, I've found this is so.

"Look," I said, "if there is a list of diseases as long as your arm, and any *one* of them can land you a diagnosis of AIDS, then how the hell can anybody be sure that the reported numbers of AIDS cases mean anything, as time passes? It could just be a collection of conditions and symptoms caused by many different things."

"Welcome to the real world," he told me. "It's not inhabited by many people."

"But," I said, "the researchers at the top of the heap claim they've *proved* that HIV is responsible for all the reported cases of AIDS and all the AIDS symptoms in the world."

The doctor laughed. "If you're asking me about how you prove a germ causes a disease, that's a whole different can of worms."

"Meaning what?"

"Meaning that researchers, first of all, have arguments among themselves about what is good proof that any germ causes a particular illness. And they like to *keep* this argument among themselves. They don't want the public to look in on it. To the public, they want to put on a good face. Like, it's no problem, we've got it all under control."

"But it's not under control?"

"What the hell do you think? Go ahead, check out the proof that HIV causes AIDS or anything else.. See what you get into."

So I did.

But first I tried to establish other situations where the symptoms of AIDS could be produced chemically, or at least without the HIV virus. I found them.

CHEMICAL AIDS

The New York doctor and I had another discussion of so-called AIDS symptoms.

"There are other drugs you should know about," he said. "Preludin and Atabrine, for example. Preludin was taken by some men in the gay bathhouse scene. It's a form of speed. If you look at the adverse reactions, you'll think you're reading a mish-mash of pre-AIDS, AIDS, and slim symptoms."

I did look up reactions to the drugs he mentioned. Any standard drug guide[1] will tell you Preludin can produce weakness, fatigue, malaise, confusion, shortness of breath, diarrhea, stomach pains, rash, bone marrow depression (immune-system components are made in the bone marrow), excessive sweating, chills, fever, suppression of appetite.

Atabrine, an antiparasitic drug used when intestinal parasites began to take a toll among gays in San Francisco, in the mid-1970s, also has a familiar list of symptoms it can bring on: diarrhea, abdominal pain, skin eruptions, hepatitis, aplastic anemia (an immunosuppressed state which gives rise to opportunistic infections), dermatitis.

"Look," this deep-throat doctor told me, "medical people who see lots of AIDS patients know that many, many of them develop certain types of infections. They have skin problems, rashes, inflammatory infections, they have fungal infections that don't go away, they have other bacterial infections. They are fatigued. They have fevers, diarrhea, shortness of breath. They're weak. They have stomach pains, they don't want to eat. The most prevalent diseases are pneumocystis pneumonia and Kaposi's sarcoma. We see all these patterns over and over. And we see a wasting away. But nobody is seriously considering that these symptoms could mainly be caused by various

---

[1]In this book, I most often used *Lippincott's Drug Facts and Comparisons* (1988).

chemicals. Nobody is seriously thinking that these symptoms could, in different people, be caused by *different combinations* of chemical factors, or by older diseases like syphilis. Well, a few people are, but the big-money boys, the people that control AIDS research grants in this country – they're not interested in these avenues of research."

I said, "I don't consider these chemicals just promising avenues. If you define a disease or a syndrome like AIDS so that it has forty symptoms, and all forty can be produced by drugs, then if the people who are sick have been taking those drugs . . . it's criminal to avoid the obvious conclusion."

I spoke to another gay man originally from San Francisco. In the 70s, he said, the drug MDA was prevalent in parts of the gay community. MDA has an amphetamine component to go along with its accent on sensuality.

"You could dance on it all night. Or you could go to the baths with it," he told me. "The only thing was, it left you depleted afterword. If you used it in quantity, which many people did, you'd take it three or four times on Friday night, and three or four times on Saturday night, once on Sunday night, maybe once during the week. That could add up to a lot of depletion.

"There was another thing. With this heavy MDA use, you wouldn't get an erection, although you'd be very turned on sexually. So in the bathhouse, for example, you'd go more toward being a sexual "bottom."[2] If you weren't already, MDA would definitely lead you in that direction, aggressively. You'd screw as many times as you could.

"Early in 1981, before there was the name AIDS, I began to notice that the gay men I knew who were dying had been using MDA, or they were MDA dealers, or friends of dealers. It was obvious to a lot of people that this was happening. Those MDA people had become depleted. They wasted away and died."

Q: I'm told a frequent combination of drugs, used during a night at the bathhouse, consisted of poppers, MDA, quaaludes and valium.

---

[2] Anal-receptive partner.

A: Valium? We'd use that to relax after sex, after we were through.

Q: You told me quaaludes became contaminated about 1980.

A: People kept track of these things all through the 70s. Yes, the reports coming back from labs where you could send drugs for analysis were not very encouraging. That was in 1980. The quaaludes contained byproducts and reagents. In other words, the underground chemists who were now making them were careless. In purifying the drug at each step of the chemical process, they weren't getting rid of all the byproducts.

Q: Quaaludes were obviously a sexual drug.

A: Best one ever made. There was a general attrition on the bathhouse scene due to the drugs. In the mid 70s, intestinal parasites became a widespread problem, too. These were serious parasites. They were terrible. They were being passed around.

Q: What drugs were you using for parasites?

A: Different ones. Lomatil, flagyl, Atabrine, Diiodoquin. The worst effects were with flagyl and Atabrine. A number of people experienced horrible feelings of malaise and depression from them. A what's-the-use-of-living feeling. People stopped taking them.

The action of these anti-parasitic drugs is very revealing, to say the least. Flagyl is known to cause a sudden overgrowth of candida in the body. It would explain some of the so-called mysterious candidiasis among gay men, which became a hallmark for the diagnosis of AIDS.

Lomotil, used to manage diarrhea, may actually aggravate diarrhea if patients have salmonella in their systems. In fact, this germ *was* present in many people, and later came to be listed as an indicator disease for AIDS. Aggravated diarrhea would lead to further dehydration, which would mean heavy loss of electrolytes, and this in turn could create "AIDS dementia" symptoms: disorientation, confusion. In addition, Lomotil does cause central nervous system reactions: malaise, depression, numbness of extremities. It exacerbates depression in patients who use barbiturates, tranquilizers, or alcohol.

The above catalog of symptoms weaves in well with what is thought to be pre-AIDS or AIDS. A mistaken diagnosis would be all too easy to make.

The other drug mentioned for parasites, diiodoquin, has a startling history under a variety of names, the most notable of which are diiodohydroxyquin, iodoquinol and vioform.

Researcher Roulette Smith[3] mentions that diiodohydroxyquin was given to Haitian boat people in the US when some of them were found to have parasites. He also indicates that the drug has been heavily marketed in Zaire and Angola. AIDS has been diagnosed, of course, in all three of these populations. The drug can cause skin rash, diarrhea, headaches, and there is some suggestion that it is toxic to DNA and is cancer-causing. What Smith calls a related antiparasitic drug, clioquinol, was implicated in a severe and widespread nervous disorder, called SMON, in Japan. Between 1962 and 1978, 8000-11000 cases were diagnosed, and at least 700 people died. Its symptoms included abdominal pain, diarrhea, paralysis, blindness, degeneration of muscles and nerves, weakness of legs (now rated an early sign of AIDS dementia), and death. Needless to say, all these symptoms can now be considered part of the AIDS complex.

The Japanese government undertook an extensive investigation of SMON, to determine its cause, and in 1978, a Japanese court ruled that clioquinol was to blame. Ciba-Geigy, which had been marketing the compound there under various names, in 200 different products, paid settlements to 1500 victims and the families of those who died. (In 1970, according to reports, Ciba-Geigy withdrew all 200 of these products from the Japanese market, and in the following year less than 40 cases of SMON were noted.)

There has been no information released from the AIDS research establishment on these antiparasitic drugs, and unfortunately epidemiologists do not readily accept the fact that people on the scene,

---

[3] See *Annals of NY Academy of Sciences*, v. 437, p. 595, 1984.

such as the man I interviewed here, know much more about what harms local people than they do.

In the following weeks, I found more evidence of "chemical AIDS." And I became more sure that, aside from a large group of wide-ranging symptoms, there was no central core to AIDS, there was no central thing which gave this list of symptoms special meaning. So for every chemical I could dig up which caused one more "AIDS symptom," I was advancing a valid explanation. To scientists who complained, "You're just finding reasons for individual symptoms, not for AIDS," I replied, "No, you fellows started all this. You assembled the massive numbers of unrelated symptoms and called them AIDS."

That wasn't a very popular comment.

CHAPTER FIVE

WHO POPPED THE POPPERS?

Shortly after our phone conversation, the New York MD sent me a letter.

". . . They're going to try to say that chemicals can't cause AIDS because they aren't immunosuppressive, they're just bad for your health. They're going to try to say they understand exactly how and exactly where HIV attacks the immune system. That's baloney.[1]

"Human immune response isn't a few pieces of tinkertoys interacting. Immunity involves the skin, for example, and the nervous system in general. Impair it and you have lowered immune response and opened doors to more infections. These are obvious known facts.

"So don't buy the idea that AIDS is some specialized attack on a special piece of the immune system and they know all about it. That's the facade they're maintaining. The truth is, they don't know. They don't know at all."[2]

The next drug I came across was familiar to some AIDS researchers. It was generally conceded that inhalant nitrites, or poppers, were harmful to one's health, but how or why . . . these issues, it seemed, could be debated for years with no answer.

Although TV news and newspapers brim over with accounts of the latest surmises about HIV, they don't discuss amyl or isobutyl or butyl nitrites. That is because press representatives at NIH and the CDC don't have a great deal to say about nitrites. The stress is on HIV. So press coverage, too, leans in the official direction, despite the

[1]See, for example, "The Acquired Immunodeficiency Syndrome: Current Status," *Yale Journal of Biology and Medicine*, 1982, p. 443, Quagliarello. It refers to immunosuppression among opiate addicts as a result of their drug intake, not AIDS.

[2]See the *New York Times*, Dec. 21, 1987, p. 1. Douglas Dietrich of the New York Medical Center told reporter Gina Kolata, "I've followed patients who've had T-cell counts of less than 10 for a year, and nothing happened to them." Conventional wisdom has it that such an apparent deficiency of immune cells should signal drastic ill-health and, in fact, is one of the clear symptoms of AIDS. Dieterich's findings suggest the current model of how AIDS specifically affects immunity is speculative.

fact that, if you had to choose between evidence suggesting an AIDS-popper link or an AIDS-HIV link, you might well take the poppers.

Inhalant nitrites have been used widely in the gay community as an orgasm-enhancer and muscle relaxer during sex, especially for anal intercourse. They have now been banned in Wisconsin, New York, and Massachusetts. California still allows them to be sold but has a law requiring warning signs to be posted at point of sale.

The multimillion dollar popper industry has managed to stay alive by classifying and selling its products as room odorizers, although under such interesting names as Hard Ware, with, for example, this slightly off-key inducement – "Never before has an aroma attracted such attention!" A May, 1985, ad in the *Advocate* showed a bottle of Hard Ware with a warning prominently printed on the neck of the bottle: WARNING: MAY BE FATAL IF SWALLOWED. SKIN IRRITANT AND SEVERE EYE IRRITANT. FLAMMABLE.

Dr. Harry Haverkos, a researcher on nitrites, formerly of the CDC, now at the National Institute on Drug Abuse, remarks: "The proven potential for cancer causing nitrosamine in bacon, for example, is probably one-millionth of the dose from inhalation of poppers."

A recent bill authored by California Congressman Mel Levine demanded full federal accounting of the dangers of poppers. In December of 1987, eight months late, the report appeared. It affirmed a policy of no-action against popper companies and offered no suggestions for regulating the nitrite drug-group.

Much earlier, on May 6, 1985, Dr. James Curran, Chief of AIDS Branch at the CDC, wrote the following letter to Hank Wilson, head of the Committee to Monitor Poppers in San Francisco.[3]

"Some of the studies (on nitrites) you cite are outdated and some are quite current. You have edited and amalgamated them skillfully...It is possible that heavy use of nitrites, or another factor correlated with such use, may contribute in some as yet undefined

---

[3] The letter was published in John Lauritsen and Hank Wilson's *Death Rush, Poppers and AIDS*, Pagan Press, New York, 1986. This book is an indispensable guide to understanding the potential harm of poppers.

way to the development of Kaposi's sarcoma in those already infected with (HIV) or who have AIDS.

"I agree that this information should be disseminated and I acknowledge the active role you have played in this effort. On the other hand, the present data do not justify an absolute 'anti-popper' campaign.

"We certainly wish to point out that no data exist to indicate that using nitrites is a safe, risk-free practice. Gay men should consider decreasing use of this substance until more data are available to assess those risks that may exist.

"Thank you for your interest in this issue."

Three years have passed since Curran wrote this letter. Whatever minor funding has subsequently gone into nitrite research, none of the dissemination of information about poppers Curran paid lipservice to has taken place. No serious attempt, at the federal health level, has been made to warn or advise against nitrites. Apparently the above piece of skillful equivocation was the limit of CDC involvement in the matter.

In the Sept.-Oct. 1984 issue of *Pharmacotherapy*, GR Newell presented this interesting short history of poppers: "Volatile nitrite in the form of amyl nitrite was used for 100 years for the treatment of angina pectoris. In spite of recognized toxicity, its use in this form was considered safe. During the 1960s, prescriptions were not required for purchase of amyl nitrite . . . and its use for recreational purposes became popular.[4] With reinstatement of the prescription requirement in 1969, non-medicinal street variety volatile nitrites were made commercially available in the form of mixtures of impure butyl and isobutyl nitrite; some of these preparations also included amyl nitrite. These products have been found to be profoundly immunosuppressive for human lymphocytes in vitro, and their byproducts when metabolized into N-nitroso compounds have been known to be highly carcinogenic in many animal species. Recreational use of inhaled volatile nitrites is prevalent among male homosexuals and

---

[4] The quantities used per person then accelerated fantastically.

compounds have been suspected as possible co-factors in Kaposi's sarcoma associated with AIDS."

Authors Lauritsen and Wilson, in *Death Rush, Poppers and AIDS*, provide further interesting groundwork. They report that Doctor Sue Watson, after sending a letter about popper-dangers to the *Journal of the American Medical Association* in 1982 – which was rejected – wrote a letter to the *Advocate*, the largest gay publication in America:

"Our studies show that amyl nitrite strongly suppressed the segment of the immune system (cellular immunity) which normally protects individuals against Kaposi's sarcoma, Pneumocystis pneumonia, herpes virus, Candida, amebiasis, and a variety of other opportunistic infections. The upshot of this research is that persons using nitrite inhalants may be at risk for development of AIDS...Publication of this letter in the *Advocate* will serve to alert the community to the health risks of using amyl nitrite. I hope you will see fit to include this information in the news section of the *Advocate*."

The letter was not answered. The Advocate did not print it.

Hank Wilson, chairman of the San Francisco-based Committee to Monitor Poppers, then got hold of another letter written to the *Advocate* by Joseph Miller, president of Great Lakes Products, Inc. Great Lakes manufactures nitrites and markets them through gay publications as room odorizers. Because the CDC had never taken any action against nitrites, and had in fact exonerated them through its policy of equivocation, Miller could expansively pen the following:

"As the largest advertiser in the Gay press, we intend to use the extensive ad space we purchase each month as the vehicle for sending a message of good health to the North American Gay communities."

Wilson and Lauritsen recount that, on April 1, 1983, Joseph Miller issued a press release titled, *U.S. Government Studies Now Indicate that Nitrite-Odorants Not Related to AIDS!* It was mentioned in the release that the assistant director of the Center for Infectious Diseases (at the CDC), James Curran, had given Miller an invitation to visit the CDC in November of 1982 –and that the CDC then told him "no association exists between nitrite-based odorants and AIDS."

Miller's press release then offered this disclaimer: "Although his (Miller's) company does not advocate the misuse of HARD-WARE® or QUICKSILVER® as inhalants, Miller says the company is greatly relieved to know that recent Government studies clearly show that such misuse poses no health hazard."

Wilson and Laurtisen report that six months later, on September 27, 1983, James Curran of the CDC sent a letter to Miller, and a copy to the *Advocate*, which never printed it. Curran didn't deny he had met with Miller at the CDC, but he was upset with Miller's attempted whitewash of popper health-dangers: "Other health hazards (than AIDS) from misuse of these drugs have been documented," Curran replied. "Your press release and advertisements in the *Advocate*[5] are misleading and misrepresent the CDC findings and their implications . . . While it is unlikely that nitrites will be implicated as the primary cause of AIDS, their role as a co-factor in some of the illnesses found in this syndrome has not been ruled out. I must insist that you discontinue the misuse and misinterpretation of CDC findings."

It is highly probable that the first five, the first fifty, the first hundred AIDS cases were all heavy inhalant nitrite users.[6]

Like other street drugs, poppers too were adulterated. Wilson and Lauritsen point out, "In 1981, the Stanford Medical Laboratories tested some samples of different brands of poppers, and found them to contain kerosene, hydrochloric acid, and sulfur dioxide, among other impurities."

A number of studies[7] have shown a link between nitrites and the development of Kaposi's sarcoma in particular. Among those diagnosed with AIDS as a result of contracting Kaposi, the overwhelm-

---

[5] I am told the *Advocate* no longer runs popper ads.

[6] See appendix to this book, "The First Five AIDS Cases." Also see "Disseminated Kaposi's Sarcoma in Homosexual Men," Friedman-Kien et al, *Annals of Internal Medicine*, June, 1982, p. 693; "Disease Manifestation among Homosexual Men with AIDS," *Sexually Transmitted Diseases*, Oct.-Dec., 1985., Haverkos et al, p. 103; "National Case-Control Study of Kaposi's Sarcoma and Pneumocystis Carinii Pneumonia in Homosexual Men: Part One, Epidemiological Results," *Annals of Internal Medicine*, August, 1983, Jaffe et al, p. 145.

[7] For example, "A Case-Control Study of Risk Factors for AIDS in San Francisco," Andrew Moss. Presented 15 April 1985 at the CDC Conference on AIDS in Atlanta.

ing majority have been gay men. It is well established that heavy nitrite use has centered in pockets of the gay community, and that its
use outside those circles, in such high dose levels, has been relatively
rare.

The question arises, how might inhalant nitrites contribute to
Kaposi's sarcoma?

One answer is that exposure of the skin to nitrites produces carcinogenic compounds (called nitrosamines). Another is that Kaposi
is not really a cancer of the blood vessels at all, that its lesions are the
results of blood vessels becoming weak and incompetent. That this
incompetency is not a malignancy, but the onset of many lesions in
many places, owing to the action of nitrites, which dialate the vessels.
This repeated action, under extremely large doses, could cause
mechanical breakdown of the blood vessels, which would result in lesions and bleeding.

When patients do die of Kaposi itself, which is not often, it is
usually the result of internal bleeding from the lesions.

CHAPTER SIX

DRUGS AND AIDS: AN INTERVIEW WITH
AN AIDS CLINIC ADMINISTRATOR

Jack True is a hynotherapist. Since 1982, he has interviewed about 600 people with AIDS. For the last year and a half, he has worked as administrator of the Natural Therapies Medical Clinic in Santa Monica, California.

He is one of several people with whom I have discussed AIDS patients' background-profiles.[1] Since published studies along this line leave out one or more important factors, the best information at present comes from people like True. What he says correlates with observations of others I've talked to.

Q: What are the most commonly held factors you've found, since 1982, in people with AIDS?

True: In *all* the people I've encountered, there's been a high level of stress – occupational, in relationships, in the way they play. These are party people, by and large. Into night life, heavy drug use, recreational and medical drugs, promiscuity.

Q: What are the percentages of gay and straight people you've seen?

A: About 70% gay, 15% bisexual, 10% straight.

Q: Of the straight people, what were the most commonly held factors?

A: Drug use, medical and recreational. Stress in family relationships. Not so much of the promiscuity. Some, but not so much.

Q: Since you started working at the Natural Therapies Clinic, would you say you've seen a representative sample of people who've been diagnosed with AIDS?

---

[1] Also see Joan McKenna's comments on background profiles in *AIDS and Syphilis-- The Hidden Link* by Harris L. Coulter, North Atlantic Books, 1987, p. 46-8. E.g., "...reports of prescribed tetracycline for 5 to 18 years, continously (among AIDS patients interviewed)."

A: I've seen very few people without education. Most of these people are professionals. Engineers, accountants, psychologists, people in show biz, restaurant people . . . The ten cases I'm giving you are the norm for what I've seen. The large drug use is there. It cries out to be ranked as the key factor. You go in different directions: This person did pain pills, that person did heavy antibiotics, another person did recreational drugs in large amounts over a long period of time. Now you put the word AIDS on top of these people and you have the effect of a powerful debilitating suggestion.

Here is my brief summary of Mr. True's ten cases.

No. 1. White male bisexual, 30's, married, with children. Candida, fungal infections. Very agitated, tense person. It turned out that, in Phoenix, he had a gay lover, and this was known only by his brother, who tried to get him certified and locked up. Main drugs he used were cocaine and alcohol. Difficult to unravel all the facts relevant to illness in this situation, because he is so secretive. Recently admitted a five-year period, in another city, when he was regularly visiting bathhouses. STDs?[2]

No. 2. 27-year-old white gay male. Well educated. Worked as a bathhouse attendant in New York for three years. Started hustling sex when he was 17. Has had Kaposi's sarcoma for three years. As a bathhouse attendant, he was usually paid in drugs for arranging rooms for customers. Has done lots of drugs since early teens. Angel dust, coke, grass, poppers, downers, quaaludes, MDA, acid, a great deal of antibiotics. Many incidents of gonorrhea. Got into the S and M lifestyle on the M side, and because he took so many drugs, he had to engage in more brutal games to feel anything because the drugs were desensitizing his body. Steady junk food diet.

No. 3. 32-year-old white gay man. Has had Kaposi's sarcoma for a little over a year. Extremely good looking. "A single blemish freaks him out." His main drug was steroids, which he took over a long period to develop more bulk and muscle. Pumped lots of iron. Eventually had an episode of pneumocystis. He smoked pot every day for five years, consistently did poppers and MDA at bathhouses.

---

[2] Sexually transmitted diseases.

Was a bottom. For twelve years, he's been taking antibiotics prophylactically, so he won't get pimples. A doctor in New Jersey started him on this regimen, which also involved cortisone and hormone creams.

No. 4. 52-year-old white gay man. Was diagnosed as pre-AIDS with swollen lymph nodes, in 1986, in London. Leads a usual kind of stressful business life. He is not as heavy a drug user as some, but does his share: booze, grass, sleeping pills on a regular basis, pain pills, mood elevators, a little speed. He is a top. Has a history of inflammatory and urethral problems.

No. 5. 23-year-old white gay man. One incident of pneumocystis. Managed to put in 18-hour work days on a regular basis. Never particularly healthy. Considerable drug-taking habits. Twenty to thirty cups of coffee every day, a history of speed, valium, grass, thorazine. Alcohol. Has had syphilis and gonorrhea, many incidents of the latter. Has taken much antibiotics.

No. 6. 34-year-old male bisexual. Emaciated, weight-loss. Lives on a total junk-food diet, shoots heroin, shoots cocaine, free bases, has a long history of gonorrhea, which has now become both front and back, and he is frequently re-infected. Much antibiotics.

No. 7. 23-year-old heterosexual. Had pneumonia, but a definitive diagnosis of pneumocystis was not made. Has also had fungal infections, while he lived in Miami. Has sex with new women 4-5 times a week. Long history of antibiotics, taken for STDs, but also to "stave off possible infections." He dealt drugs in Miami and used coke, speed, downers.

No. 8. 44-year-old white gay man from Denmark. Somewhat promiscuous. 25-year, heavy alcoholic. Recently joined AA. Long history of depression. After an automobile accident, had a major operation and a transfusion. Did not recover well, and began losing weight.

No. 9. 54-year-old semi-retired male. Bisexual. Has had candida, other fungal infections. 20 years of promiscuous sex, much of it in bathhouses. Has had immunotoxic medical drug therapy for a cancer, also has a history of hepatitis B and STDs. Took many gammaglobulin[3] shots. 5-10 years of amphetamines.

No. 10. 35-year-old heterosexual. Has had both pneumocystis and severe herpes, hepatitis A, B, while living in Europe. Has taken many gammaglobulin shots, had has several STD episodes. Shoots heroin regularly, is quite promiscuous. Has used alcohol every day for six years (averages five drinks a day).

This is not to suggest that there are no puzzling cases of diagnosed AIDS, in which the immunosuppressive factors are harder to find. Those hard-to-understand situations, as well as others, may involve syphilis. But again, as I mentioned, the above 10 cases are normal in the experience of, not just Mr. True, but many clinicians and therapists.

The combination of many drugs and STDs is common. In other words, immunosuppression *already exists* from factors having nothing to do with the HIV virus.

---

[3] A blood component which contains many antibodies.

CHAPTER SEVEN

YEARS OF ANTIBIOTICS: MORE ON CHEMICAL AIDS

Antibiotics, by many accounts, have been overused tremendously in certain pockets of the American gay community, in the last fifteen years. In this, such gays represent an extreme example of general overuse, particularly in hospitals. From reports of several clinicians who interview people with AIDS, there are cases where these people have taken antibiotics for ten years, continuously.

This practice started taking off in the 60s. A gay man, going to, say, Puerto Rico on vacation might ask his doctor for a script, for antibiotics, because he wasn't sure he could get one in Puerto Rico. His doctor would write one out.

Prophylactic dosing continued when the same gay man, back in New York, would anticipate going to the baths on the weekend. He would load up on tetracycline, just to make sure he would be okay if he ran into gonorrhea bacteria. And so on and so forth, until, among some people, popping antibiotics became a daily regimen, a habit, as San Francisco physiologist Joan McKenna says, "against the possibility of a pimple."

Overprescription of antibiotics has two principal effects. It creates antibiotic-resistant germs which then become harder to treat, and it upsets in the patient's body the balance of microbes which has been established over the course of evolution.

Physicians, then faced with antibiotics having no effect on their patients' infections – and not realizing that the cause is genetic resistance which has been built up by those germs to antibiotics – can in some cases jump the gun and assume the patients are so immunedepressed that "drugs don't work anymore."

Leading to false diagnoses of AIDS.

A patient, through overuse of antibiotics, carries around with him an imbalance of germs in which harmful micro-organisms have gained the upper hand in territories of the body in which their natural competitors have been drugged out of existence.

Two instances of this are salmonella and candida albicans.

Both are specifically listed as grounds for a diagnosis of AIDS on the September 4, 1987, CDC definition of AIDS, even though these infections can clearly develop for no other reason than antibiotic-abuse.

Other similar instances are streptococcus, Proteus and Pseudomonas. Any of these alone could be defined as AIDS.[1] You may, if you wish, rely on the wisdom of your doctor to know about the strange imbalancing effects of antibiotic overprescription – but the facts are that most physicians are unaware of, or ignore, that potentially important element of disease in 1988.

1. In some areas of the third world where AIDS cases are reported, antibiotic use has grown tremendously. Prescriptions are rarely necessary. The drugs are sold over the counter and then shot or swallowed.

2. One of the most toxic antibiotics, chloramphenicol, whose use is carefully monitored in the US, is shipped to Brazil, parts of Africa, and Mexico where, bought over the counter, it can suppress immune systems by harming bone marrow.

3. Some antibiotics inhibit protein-synthesis and are thus toxic (immunosuppressive). The universally used tetracycline falls into this category.

4. It is probable that certain bacteria are useful to us because, without being harmful, they "exercise" our immune systems and keep them in good scavenging shape. Antibiotic overuse can demolish these useful strains.

5. Beneficial skin bacteria act as a kind of immune system of their own, protecting us against Staph, Strep, Neisseria (meningitis, gonorrhea), Clostridium, Cornebacterium. Again, antibiotics can

---

[1] They fall under the category of "other bacterial infections."

sweep the deck clean and rid us of these "immunizing" helpful bacteria.

     6. As previously mentioned, several clinicians and Joan McKenna, a San Francisco physiologist, report, from many interviews of gay AIDS patients, extensive long-term use of antibiotics (prophylactic) for possible STD infections – *10-15 years of more or less continuous usage.* One can infer that these men's bodies are filled with antibiotic-resistant strains of bacteria. Also that these resistant bacteria are being passed around in dense quantities in areas of the gay community. Doctors are naturally baffled by the failure of many types of antibiotics to put a dent in these bacterial infections. An AIDS myth begins: Bacterial infections and their unmanageability are said to be entirely the result of underlying immune-suppression from the HIV virus.

     7. Some British strains of staph bacteria (called "80") seem to be more powerfully infecting than previous staph types. 80s are all antibiotic-resistant. There is the possibility that some bacteria *strengthen* because of antibiotic treatment, beyond the fact that they become harder to subdue with treatment.

     8. Hemophilus b, a microbe involved in pneumonia as well as other illness (pneumonitis, by CDC definition, is sufficient for a diagnosis of AIDS), has increasingly grown resistant to antibiotics. This process probably began in the 1950s and has continued to the present.[2]

     I believe that a physician who writes scripts for antibiotics casually and continously, as "prevention," should be liable for serious criminal charges. If the Centers for Disease Control want to perform a good deed that will indeed control disease, the drafting of such a bill for Congressional approval would be in order, and would cause an immediate upsurge in medical knowledge to course through the professional community.

     It's worth adding at this point that Dr. James O. Mason, head of the CDC, was a Mormon bishop, a quite high-ranking official in a faith which professes a strong belief in preventive medicine. In fact,

---

[2] See the excellent *When Antibiotics Fail,* by Marc Lappe, North Atlantic Books, 1986. Some of the basics of antibiotic-abuse recounted here are derived from Lappe's account.

the church's foreign medical missionary program, once headed by Dr. Mason, stressed preventive-health advice in the Third World.

It's surprising that the scandalous role of antibiotic overprescription in both causing disease to appear and to resist treatment has not been handled with more firmness by Dr. Mason.

What happens when a person ingests antibiotics on a scale never envisioned, inhales enough amyl and butyl nitrite to float a continent, and is infected a dozen times in two years with various strains of gonorrhea or syphilis? The answer may well be, his immune system dives into oblivion, and otherwise benign microbes in his body, such as pneumocystis protozoa, begin to erupt in virulent ways, ways we have come to call, irrelevantly, AIDS.

CHAPTER EIGHT

PESTICIDES AND DRUG DUMPING IN THE THIRD WORLD: IS IT AIDS?

As David Weir and Mark Shapiro note in their landmark book, *Circle of Poison* (Institute for Food and Development Policy, San Francisco, 1981), parathion, a major killer among pesticides, was developed first by Nazi scientists as a weapon during WWII. After minor alteration, it became a pesticide; in its present form, it is still 60 times more toxic to humans than DDT. It is widely distributed in the Third World.

Phosvel, a pesticide outlawed in the U.S., was marketed in the Third World in the 1970s, and may still be trading in Latin America. Its victims are called "zombies." They die slowly and agonizingly, with paralysis and asphyxiation coming at the end.[1] Field workers who suffer weight loss and an increasing inability to move should not be assumed, by researchers a continent away, to be suffering from a virus.

A Nairobi professor visited a pesticide plant in Kenya in the late 1970s. The product BHC was being made there, and protection of workers against its toxic effects was nil. "The workers' eyes were all sunken," the professor reported, "and they all looked like they had TB."[2] When these workers get sick they are fired.

When selling dangerous pesticides from the West to the Third World is frowned on or outlawed by their own governments, Western corporations sometimes circumvent these regulations by setting up so-called formulator plants in Third World countries. Ingredients for the banned pesticides are shipped separately to these plants and combined there, usually under no rules of safety. The worst of these

---

[1] *Circle of Poison.*
[2] Forms of TB are now listed as AIDS indicator-diseases.

plants are small local operations, run like "whiskey stills." In Brazil, there are perhaps 8000 such backyard chemists.

With Brazil suffering from a large upswing in various traditional diseases, as well as from endemic malnutrition, a chemical infusion of 8000 unshielded toxic pollutors could easily create pockets of new wasting-away diseases. With actual causes overlooked and ignored, the faddish medical pronouncement could certainly be AIDS.

Prospects for the future of pesticides? The United Nations Food and Agriculture Organization (FAO) predicts that by the year 2000, 67% of the seeds used in underdeveloped countries will be "improved." This means they will be altered to yield more production, but will also be more vulnerable to pests. Therefore, they will require more pesticides. Weir and Shapiro indicate that pesticide companies are in fact, through buy-outs, starting to corner the market on global seed businesses; the creation of seeds which *require* fertilizers and pesticides is the work of these parent companies.

Weir and Shapiro's Table of "Recent North American Seed Company Acquisitions" leaves no doubt that chemistry for better living is the operating motto of some very major corporations. Prominent pharmaceutical names on the list of those taking over seed companies are: Upjohn, Sandoz, Pfizer, Monsanto, and Ciba-Geigy.

If you add in the fact that roughly 40% of the antibiotics sold in the US goes to the livestock industry to be included automatically in commercial feeds, you begin to see an obvious community of interest that runs very deep: pesticides, pharmaceuticals, agriculture.

It is difficult to trace specific pesticides from the U.S. and Europe through to use in, say, African countries or Brazil. The general rule of thumb is, the *most toxic* pesticides are used in the Third World, and there they are used (and formulated) with frightening disregard for safety. This is due to a lack of laws, and also to the fact that label-warnings printed on containers in English have no meaning for most of the people who handle these poisons.

In books such as *Circle of Poison*, we get glimpses of field workers suffering extreme effects from casual contact with these substances.

A worker in Guatemala might use old Coke bottles to apportion amounts of parathion for local farmers. No protection, no seals on the bottles, no labels, no warnings.

Consider the case of Phosvel, recounted in *Circle*. In 1976, the Texas plant which manufactured the pesticide had to close because workers there were developing central nervous system problems. "Fellow workers dubbed them 'Phosvel Zombies' because they lost their coordination, and their ability to work, talk and think clearly."

A scandal developed. Workers filed suit against the manufacturer, Velsicol. Nevertheless, the company continued to sell the product in the Third World. This, despite the fact that in 1971, in Egypt, "a widely publicized Phosvel epidemic . . . killed over 1,000 water buffalo and an unknown number of peasants. The victims died a slow and agonizing death, gradually paralyzed until they asphyxiated."

Phosvel belongs to the class of pesticides called organophosphates. Here is a list[3] of symptoms which can be caused by organophosphates: headache, dizziness, flu-like symptoms, excessive sweating, difficulties walking, diarrhea, many skin problems, delayed nerve disease.

Headache is now listed by the World Health Organization as a significant symptom of "early HIV disease."[4] Many researchers state that HIV causes a *mild flu-like episode* soon after exposure. *Night sweats* are taken as a sign of Pre-AIDS. *Leg weakness* is considered an early symptom of AIDS dementia. *Diarrhea* can be a sign of pre-AIDS and also a major symptom of AIDS in the Third World. AIDS patients often present *numerous skin rashes and skin problems*. *Nerve disease* is said to be the reason for AIDS dementia.

In other words, the symptoms of exposure to organophosphates read like listed symptoms for AIDS.

---

[3] This list and the following lists of symptoms are taken from *Fruits of Your Labor, A Guide to Pesticide Hazards for California Field Workers*, by Sidney Weinstein, Labor Occupational Health Program, University of California, Berkeley, 1984.

[4] See *Western Journal of Medicine*, December, 1987, "AIDS, A Global Perspective," for a definition of early HIV disease.

There are at least three other major classes of pesticides: organochlorines; nitrophenols; and chlorophenoxy herbicides. As you can see, their symptoms likewise are mirrors of AIDS and Pre-AIDS symptoms.

Organochlorines: skin irritation, rash, nervous system disorders, weakness, appetite and weight loss.

Nitrophenols: sweating, headache, fever, skin rash, weight loss.

Chlorophenoxy herbicides: skin rash, muscular weakness, nerve disease. Some of these herbicides are contaminated with dioxin, one of the most toxic substances yet encountered.

The pesticides aldrin and dieldrin, both restricted in the U.S., are dumped into Africa and Latin America, along with lindane and DDT; WHO estimates 5000 deaths occur per year and 500,000 people are poisoned in those areas of the world from contact with the pesticides.

DDT, acccording to *Circle of Poison*, banned for crops in the U.S. in 1972, continued to be turned out by Montrose Chemical, which, ten years later, informed the Environmental Protection Agency that it had sold the pesticide to 21 foreign sources in 1980.

DDT had once been thought to be a boon, because it greatly reduced malaria by killing mosquitos. But now, internationally, malaria has come back with a vengeance, despite an assault with larger and larger amounts of DDT and other preparations. The new strains of mosquitos are resistant to several pesticides simultaneously and are causing, for example, in Sri Lanka, 2 million cases of malaria a year. At one earlier point, the count had shrunk to 23 cases a year there.

But now, with the mosquitos having developed resistances, there is the double problem of malaria[5] and highly toxic pesticide-use, without success, to wipe out these insects. Although non-toxic methods are being introduced (e.g., sterile male mosquitos), pesticide manufacturers haven't by any means let go of this lucrative market.

---

[5] Malaria is generally on the rise in the Third World. Some researchers say it causes the AIDS blood test to register falsely positive.

There are, of course, also dangerous drugs which are sold in the Third World by Western pharmaceutical firms.[6]

These drugs can produce immunosuppression-leading-to-opportunistic-infections – the pattern ascribed to AIDS. Yet they are completely written out of the AIDS disease-equation by US federal health agencies.

Tetracycline, the antibiotic which can damage the liver, as well as teeth and bones, and should not be taken at all by very young children, is commonly sold over the counter throughout the Third World. No prescription necessary. Physician's references in countries like Nicaragua, Brazil, and Argentina don't mention the side effects. Manufacturers? Dow, Pfizer, Dumex, Lepatit, Lederle. An international cast, which is the case with most of these drugs.

Squibb makes a vitamin preparation called Verdivitone, which is sold in Bangladesh over the counter. In that country, 50-60% of the people have liver problems. Verdivitone is 17% alcohol, definitely not recommended for people with liver disease. Local ads discuss its capacity to produce "vitality and energy."

The pharmaceutical giant, Ciba-Geigy, markets a painkiller called Cibalgin which is available, again, over the counter, in Mozambique. It contains aminopyrine, banned in the U.S. and parts of Europe because it has been linked to blood disorders. People using it have died from the opportunistic infections breaking out on top of their sudden anemias.[7] Cibalgin can also cause vomiting, kidney problems, and reddish lumps on the body.

Chloramphenicol, mentioned earlier, is manufactured by Parke Davis, McKesson, Boehringer, and Beacon. Having caused fatalities and very serious anemias, it is another drug which gets the full promotional treatment by foreign subsidiaries of the drug majors in the Third World.

---

[6] This information on drugs available in the Third World has been gathered from many observers, including representatives of Oxfam, a European-based hunger-relief organization. See *Bitter Pills*, Dianna Melrose, Oxfam publishers, 1982; and *Pills, Pesticides and Profits*, edited by Ruth Norris, North River Press, 1982.

[7] Anemia is basically an immune disorder which does what AIDS is said to do. It permits the outbreak of opportunistic infections. Its effects are, thus, indistinguishable from what is called AIDS.

Perhaps 20% of top pharmaceutical corporations' sales are made in the Third World. Total figure? Around $20 billion a year.

Hoechst of West Germany produces dipyrone, a pain reliever, which is sold over the counter in Brazil and throughout Africa. It can also cause anemia – and underlying immune suppression – and that is why it is banned in the U.S.

In Africa, there are 30 preparations listed in physician's guides which contain dipyrone or aminopyrine, mentioned above. They are touted in these guides as "analgesics for minor conditions."[8]

One certainly can't ignore the infant formula deaths either, in which diarrhea and malnutrition[9] have been linked to infant-preparations manufactured by Abbott, American Home Products, Nestle, and Bristol-Meyers. In 1980, it was estimated that *one million infant deaths per year* in the Third World were connected to the baby formulas and the absence of mother's milk.

In light of this sketch of pesticide and drug use in the Third World, it is revealing to read the latest WHO interpretation of a proper diagnosis of AIDS, as indicated by Drs. Piot and Colebunders, in "AIDS, a Global Perspective," released by WHO and published in the *Western Journal of Medicine,* December 1987. In diagnosing AIDS, the authors celebrate "the elimination of the requirement of the absence of other causes of immunodeficiency." In plain English, no longer it is necessary to scrutinize the pati nt and see where his immune-compromised condition comes from. It's SOP to overlook a multitude of sins and say, simply, *AIDS.*

This amazing WHO guideline implies that from now on, all human immunosuppression will be laid at the door of the HIV virus. No newspaper or television network has noticed this bizarre turn of events or has chosen to pursue it as a major scandal.

---

[8] A UCLA political scientist told me that, in the mid-1970s, he personally saw, in Zaire, prescription drugs from the West being sold in marketplaces, outdoors, in 80-degree weather. Many of the drugs had obviously spoiled, and the dosing by consumers followed no sensible pattern.

[9] Malnutrition is, by far, the most common cause of immune suppression in the world.

CHAPTER NINE

ENTER AZT

One drug which has immunosuppressive effects is the single medical preparation licensed to treat people diagnosed with AIDS, so it is an important substance: AZT.

A payoff of being diagnosed as antibody-positive[1] to the HIV virus is that a patient becomes a candidate for treatments of the moment. Even though he has no symptoms, doctors will begin urging that he take AZT. A recent *New York Times* [2] front-page story detailed the perverse twist physicians have recently applied in this regard.

Instead of only giving AZT to the desperately ill, as was the intent when the FDA licensed it, doctors in large numbers have taken it upon themselves to write scripts for AZT for their patients *who have no symptoms*.

At an Institute of Medicine AIDS conference held in Washington in September, 1987, William Hazeltine, chief of pharmacology at the Dana-Farber Cancer Institute in Boston, suggested an even wider possible use for AZT. Give it to people considered at high-risk for AIDS even though they *don't* test positive for HIV. Give the drug to them as a preventive step.

For prevention, use a drug, AZT, which damages bone marrow, the place where raw material for immune-cells are turned out; a drug which causes severe anemia.

Dr. Jonathan Mann, AIDS Director for the World Health Organization, on October 20, 1987, gave a special talk to the U.N. General Assembly: "Remarkable progress has been made towards treatment of AIDS virus infection. A single drug, zidovudine, also called AZT, has been shown to be effective in the treatment of some categories of

---

[1] Simply means "tested positive for exposure to HIV."
[2] Dec. 21, 1987, "Doctors Stretch Rules on AIDS Drugs," p. 1.

AIDS; although AZT has important side effects and is quite expensive ($8,000-10,000 per year per patient), it does prolong the life of persons with AIDS . . . Recently, important trials were started to see if AZT, or other drugs, can block the progression to AIDS in healthy AIDS virus-infected people. The personal and public health benefits of such protection against AIDS would be enormous."

"Blocking the progression" of HIV in healthy people, which is what Mann feels may soon be possible with AZT, would in the Third World, amount to a death sentence for many who are already suffering chronic immune-suppression owing to malnutrition. Death, not cure, is often the result of administering highly toxic drugs to the chronically undernourished.

Lippincott's *Drug Facts and Comparisons* (1988) has a number of warnings about AZT. The drug is often associated with blood toxicity, including severe anemia requiring transfusions. "Significant anemia . . . may require a dose interruption until evidence of (bone) marrow recovery is observed."

In concert with other drugs like pentamidine and acyclovir, both used for AIDS opportunistic infections, AZT toxicity could be *increased*, Lippincott's cautions. With acyclovir, there have been two reports of AZT induced neurotoxicity: profound lethargy and seizures.

For patients who have liver or kidney problems, Lippincott's states that there may be a "greater risk of toxicity from (AZT)." Many AIDS patients do, in fact, have liver complications.

A July 23rd, 1987, *New England Journal of Medicine* report indicated that out of 140 patients taking AZT in a controlled trial, "21% . . . required multiple red-cell transfusions." In a drug which is supposed to halt temporarily the spread of AIDS, its attack point is immune-cells. The *New England Journal* study goes on to say that "serious adverse effects, particularly bone marrow suppression, were observed."

Molecular biologist Peter Duesberg remarks, "AZT is very, very destructive to healthy cells. No doubt, it's a dangerous drug."

In the October 19, 1987 issue of the *New York Native*, John Lauritsen reviewed the FDA trial of AZT which resulted in its early

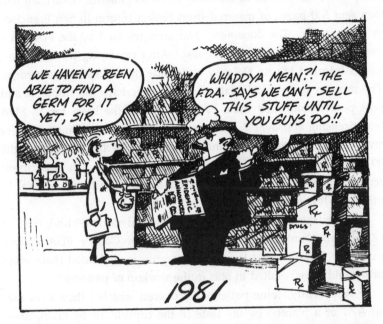

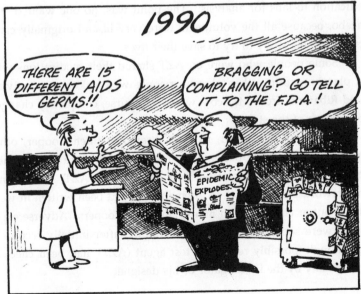

"compassionate" release to seriously ill AIDS patients. Lauritsen had been sent 500 pages of material from Project Inform in San Francisco on those trials. The documents had been released by the FDA on a Freedom of Information Act request. After reviewing these records, Project Inform's Martin Delaney had made the following assessment: "The multi-center clinical trials of AZT are perhaps the sloppiest and most poorly controlled trials ever to serve as the basis for an FDA drug licensing approval . . . causes of death (among volunteers) were never verified. Despite this and a frightening record of toxicity, the FDA approved AZT in record time, granting a treatment (recommendation) in less than five days and full pharmaceutical licensing in less than six months."

Lauritsen indicates that the controlled double-blind trial of AZT became "unblinded"[3] very quickly. Ellen Cooper, FDA analyst, is quoted: "The fact that the treatment groups unblinded themselves early could have resulted in bias in the workup of patients."

Apparently, some patients discovered whether they were taking AZT or a placebo by the taste of the capsule, or by taking their medication to labs for analysis. The point was, no one wanted the placebo, because all the volunteers were very ill and originally came forward for the study to try to save their lives.

Some people who were on AZT shared their medications with the placebo group, other placebo people were taking an antiviral called Ribavirin, from Mexico – which, of course, completely changed the outcome of the study.

Lauritsen discovered, from FDA analyst Ellen Cooper, other improprieties. Lists of patients' symptoms which were kept in their records, in order to determine their reactions to AZT, were sometimes reworked at a later date. Items which had been written in were crossed out or changed with no explanation. Cooper: "Adverse experiences were sometimes crossed out months after initially recorded, even though 'possibly related to test agent (AZT)' had been checked off originally by the investigator or his designee."

---

[3] Volunteers discovered whether they were taking AZT or a placebo.

Cooper mentions that an FDA inspector found such drastic improprieties at one AZT test center that she recommended that center, out of the twelve used, be "excluded from the analysis of the multicenter trial."[4]   At this point, three months after the study had been closed down, some attempt was made to re-evaluate what had been going on at all 12 of the AZT test-centers, but it was too late.

The AZT trial was important because it showed that the mortality of the volunteers on placebos was much higher than the AZT group. On that basis, the trial was cut short and AZT was distributed to doctors for prescribing to their ill AIDS patients.

Lauritsen, however, points out that "the death rate in the placebo group is shockingly high," and it is hard to understand why. After the trial was over, people who had been on the placebo were allowed to go on AZT openly. From this point on, the death rate of these people began to rise from the level which had occurred during the 17-week controlled trial. Also, other AZT studies which had been done previously showed a significantly *higher* death rate for those volunteers ill with AIDS *who had taken AZT*.

Harvey Chernov, an FDA analyst who looked over the pharmacological data on AZT, recommended that the drug not be approved for release.

Nevertheless, the drug was released, and it is now being prescribed loosely by many physicians for their patients who have no symptoms.

AZT attacks the immune-cells where it is speculated that HIV is doing damage. Although AZT tends slightly to favor, as a target, viruses to healthy cells, in practice it kills many healthy immune-cells.

This is the drug which is currently being touted for use as a preventive, globally, against AIDS.

A front-page article in the December 21, 1987, *New York Times* spells out the AZT scandal underway: "Defying official recommendations, a growing number of doctors who treat carriers of

---

[4] Dr. Joseph Sonnabend, former editor of *AIDS Research*, privately analyzed the AZT trials recently, and he also concluded that they were badly mismanaged.

the AIDS virus are prescribing a powerful, potentially toxic drug even before patients develop serious signs of the disease. . . Every one of more than a dozen AIDS physicians and health authorities interviewed said the practice of prescribing AZT to patients without symptoms has become widespread in recent months, as the drug, once scarce, became readily available."

The article goes on to say some doctors are alarmed that a drug which had been licensed for very narrow use, with extremely ill people, has now gotten out of hand and is being prescribed much more casually.

Dr. Itzhak Brook, who had chaired the FDA committee that originally permitted the licensing of AZT, said the wide, careless prescribing of the drug "was just what I was afraid of."

About 10,000 Americans are now taking AZT. Some of the doctors prescribing it to patients with no symptoms say they are doing so after making inferences from these patients' blood tests, which show low counts of T-cells. But there is debate over what T-cell numbers constitute immune problems.

Douglas Dieterich of the New York Medical Center told *New York Times* reporter Gina Kolata, "I've followed patients who've had T-cell counts of less than 10 for a year, and nothing happened to them." Conventional wisdom has it that a count less than 200 spells serious trouble.

A Dr. William Siroty of New York City told Kolata that he gave AZT to healthy patients who were "virus carriers" (antibody-positive) if they wanted the drug. He said they "feel better knowing they're doing something about it (HIV)."

Indeed.

An HIV-positive patient was told by his doctor he ought to start on AZT; the patient wrote him the following letter. A copy was sent to me:

"I want you to know that I cannot accept this prescription. I do not accept that my only hope is to somehow restrict the action of the HIV virus by ingesting a substance that attacks a central reservoir of my immune system.

"I have seen people with AIDS who experience a resurgence from AZT, and I won't even try to argue that some of that has to do with the placebo affect. I am interested in the long run, however, which is to say, *my life*. If I felt passive, that there was nothing I could do on my own, that no guerilla clinic might suggest a helpful compound that was less toxic than AZT, that I couldn't somehow improve my state of health, then I might say, all right, give me the AZT.

"But since I have hope, since I have a future, I don't want to wreck my immunity further with this drug. It seems to me the drug is a perfect reflection of the medical attitude toward AIDS: A dangerous poison against an invariably fatal disease. I don't believe in that 'invariably fatal' tag, and my reasons, which I won't go into here, are more than just pipe-dreams. I frankly believe that, in the AIDS equation, we, who are diagnosed with it, are considered the expendable ones.

"I am not expendable. Maybe in another cause, but not in some fabled war against a disease. Rising adrenaline among research professionals and their new grant-monies are making the medical troops and their line officers so happy . . ."

CHAPTER TEN

MALNUTRITION AIDS

I continued to find chemicals that could produce AIDS symptoms. But I also came across other factors which could cause these symptoms. Like chemicals, they had nothing to do with the fabled HIV virus. The most important one was starvation, long-term chronic malnutrition.

It can occur on one level among junkies, it can occur on an entirely different scale among people of the Third World.

Malnutrition is recognized as the single largest source of immune-suppression in the world.

For example – here is Maxime Seligmann et al, writing in the *New England Journal of Medicine*, November 15, 1984, volume 311, p. 1289: "The commonest cause of T-cell immunodeficiency[1] worldwide is protein-calorie malnutrition. Malnourished children have defects in macrophage[2] and T-cell function accompanied by . . . an increased susceptibility to infections. These effects are particularly marked in malnourished children with measles, an infection that itself causes T-cell anergy. Bacterial superinfection in these children is a major cause of serious disease and death."

RH Gray of the Johns Hopkins School of Public Health, published a 1983 study (*AJPH*, Nov. 1983, p. 1332) on protein calorie malnutrition (PCM): "There is a similarity between the immune deficiency, multiple infections, and severe weight loss seen in AIDS patients, and the association of protein calorie malnutrition with re-

---

[1] T-cell immunodeficiency is said to be a hallmark of AIDS.
[2] Attack on macrophages is the latest speculation on how the HIV virus is causing harm.

duced resistance to infection observed in malnourished children, particularly in the Third World.

"Both AIDS patients and children with PCM suffer from multiple opportunistic infections of viral, bacterial, parasitic and mycotic origin. AIDS patients have an increased incidence of Kaposi's sarcoma and diffuse undifferentiated B-cell lymphomas histologically similar to Burkitt's lymphoma. These tumors are also observed among children and young adults in East Africa, where PCM is a common condition."

By suppressing the immune system, severe malnutrition can, in fact, cause all of the indicator diseases and infections which are now thought of as AIDS-associated.

The current definitions of AIDS in the Third World now accept, by and large, three symptoms as central to AIDS: weight-loss of 10% or more (wasting away), chronic diarrhea, and chronic fever.[3]

These are *also* signs of chronic malnutrition. Diarrhea, through bringing on severe dehydration, is *traditionally* one of three largest killers in the world. This is nothing new.

The reason these three symptoms are being used as front-line indicators of AIDS involves widespread lack of lab testing facilities in Third World countries. Doctors are meant to use these indicators to do fast, on-the-spot diagnoses of AIDS. In such a situation, numbers of AIDS cases will skyrocket, and a hidden equality will be established between AIDS and hunger.

A paper published in *Nutrition and Cancer* (1985, vol. 7, p. 85-91, Chlebowski) points out a few down-to-earth facts about hunger. Chlebowski indicates that, "In studies of children in developing countries, mortality rates progressively increased from less than 1% in well-nourished children to as much as 18% in the severely malnourished population, with most deaths resulting from infections."

"Malnutrition-associated adverse effects on the cellular immune system," he continues, "include a decrease in the total number of T-lymphocytes . . . demonstrating a significant reduction princi-

---

[3] See *Lancet* October 24, 1987, "A Proposed Clinical Case Definition for AIDS in Africa."

pally of the T-helper lymphocyte population (this is seen in AIDS and is one of its immunologic hallmarks – author)."

Finally, citing another researcher, Chlebowski says, "Based on observations of pneumocystis carinii pneumonia infections in malnourished children in Haiti, Gondsmit proposed that malnutrition with concomitant herpes virus infection could give rise to symptoms that are indistinguishable from AIDS."

Africa Recovery, a UN periodical, examines the food situation in parts of Africa in its December 1987 issue. For the 15 sub-Saharan nations, cereal food aid needs – and all 15 have needs above and beyond what they grow – will not be met by outside pledges of food so far confirmed for 1988, with only two exceptions (Swaziland and Somalia).

The worst situations exist in Ethiopia and Mozambique.

In 1987, aggregate grain production in Africa as a whole fell by 15%.

115,110 tons of food for refugees were still needed for 1988, and there were no pledged sources as yet for this amount, as of December 1987.

Civil strife in the southern Sudan; cassava crop failure in Malawi; drought in pockets of Zambia, Uganda, and Zimbabwe; a sixth consecutive year of drought in Botswana; these are the less difficult situations. The major problems are in Ethiopia, Angola, and Mozambique. Another famine looms in Ethiopia. There is war in Angola and Mozambique.

In Angola, there has been large-scale destruction of health facilities. A UN interagency mission reported, "The remaining operational facilities are heavily taxed by the constantly expanding numbers of traumatized, mutilated, and seriously ill people, including numerous orphans or abandoned children." This, in addition to the reported "poor nutritional status of much of the rest of the population. Increasing population densities in the cities combined with inadequate water and sanitation systems, have favored the resurgence of highly infectious diarrheal and water born diseases, such as cholera, of which there was a major outbreak in the capital last May and June (1987)."[4]

Angola now receives outside food aid in order to survive. Many farmers, Frances Moore Lappe reports, have left their fields, because they are seeded with mines by rebels. In some areas, twenty to thirty percent of the children are suffering from malnutrition. Several hundred thousand adults are also on the verge of what could be called chronic malnutrition. (See *Betraying the National Interest*, Lappe, Schurman, and Danaher, Grove Press, 1987.)

The UN states that infant mortality has risen considerably. Listen to these figures. Of 416,000 children born in Angola each year, about 60,000 die in their first year and 100,000 die before the age of five.

The World Bank rates Zaire as the fifth poorest nation in the world. More than a third of its people die of malnutrition.

There is a long-standing international effort underway to solve problems of crop production, on many levels, in African countries. Over time, despite famine, drought, and political struggles, some of these programs are taking hold and succeeding. One question is, what stop-gap measures can be instituted on a consistent basis, into the next century, which will guarantee food to make up for shortfalls and will feed starving people?

That leads to two other worn-out questions. Is there a way of re-channeling the distribution of the world's food to feed the starving? And if this could be accomplished, what would be the consequences? The United States at present supports the World Bank and contributes money to it, a fraction of which is used in agriculture programs in the Third World. But what about the glut of food produced here now, which our farmers are paid not to sell? What would happen if our surpluses were used in Africa on a *huge* scale, directly?

That question of course embroils one immediately in political scenarios and a web of agendas held by various nations. There is no

---

[4] The latest rumblings are that outbreaks of cholera and TB will be co-opted as "AIDS diseases." Attributing such illness and misery to the HIV virus will accomplish only one thing: inflation of AIDS case numbers, leading to the sale of pharmaceuticals.

quick answer, but one of the principle rejoinders used to argue down massive food redistribution is the premise: If you feed starving people they survive, reproduce, and the population expands again, giving you new problems of starvation. And if you solve this new level of hunger, you face yet a new population increase, and so on, until the resources of the world are exhausted. But a number of studies reject this image: they maintain that with the building up of infrastructure, the birthrate in an area goes *down*.

A premise about the impossibility of feeding the world is a short step from saying, Then some of the people alive now *should* die, for the sake of us all; it is Nature's way; by interfering with the ebbs and flows we would create a more wretched world. And by this kind of reasoning, AIDS is seen as just another of Nature's plagues which from time to time water the tree of life.

A respected virologist told me exactly this several months ago. For him, there was really nothing one could do about AIDS except watch it decimate people and then, by itself, die out.

This is yet another thread in the logic that starts with the assumption that AIDS is one thing around the world, from one cause, with one invariably fatal result. The truth is, AIDS is not a single illness, it is an international operation, a business, a bureacracy. It is, in the Third World, a way of substituting harmful medical drugs for what is needed: food.

With AIDS, an attempt is being made to reduce varieties of suffering and political conflict and starvation and chemical abuse to a single entity. Since that viral entity, HIV, is sensational and frightening, it satisfies the desire not to think, not to learn, not to find out what is happening in a world of troubles.

It is also easier to dump corrosive medical drugs and pesticides on the Third World than to face up to their widening toxic effect on people. Easier to call their symptoms AIDS.

AIDS is like a horror movie made by two twenty-four-year olds who grew up in Los Angeles and learned all they know from 5000 movies they saw in Westwood.

As *The Andromeda Strain* it was entertaining as hell, but as real life it is an unqualified disaster.

CHAPTER ELEVEN

A CASE STUDY IN CONFUSION: AIDS
IN UGANDA

What happens when you try to paint a portrait of an area said to have AIDS, and you find, instead, a combination of drugs, pesticides, starvation, older diseases, and other environmental factors, *all* capable of causing immunosuppression, all capable of producing the symptoms of what is called AIDS? What happens is, if you want to satisfy your medical peers, if you want to win research grant monies, you overlook the anomalies and say it's all AIDS. If you don't, you admit the picture is diverse and confused. You face facts. You lose grants.

In Brazil, for example, a nation said to be seething with under-reported AIDS cases, they are now looking at studies which show that in the northeast, a new generation is being born. These children have smaller frames and smaller heads, because of chronic malnourishment of previous generations.

In Brazil, as in Africa, sweetheart deals are cut with multinationals who come in from abroad, loggers and cattle ranchers and agribusiness-types. The governments over there give these corporations terrific subsidies and tax-breaks, so that wood can be cut and food can be grown for export back to the industrialized world.

This involves tearing apart rain-forests. When you take the upper canopy off a rain forest, the malaria mosquitos which drone about up there come down to ground. They breed in new standing water created by big tire tracks and big shovels. They fly indoors at night. Malaria then expands by a sizeable degree.

Certain flies breed in increasing amounts in rivers which are jammed up because of logs from the lumber companies. These flies carry a parasite which causes river blindness. If you haven't already,

71

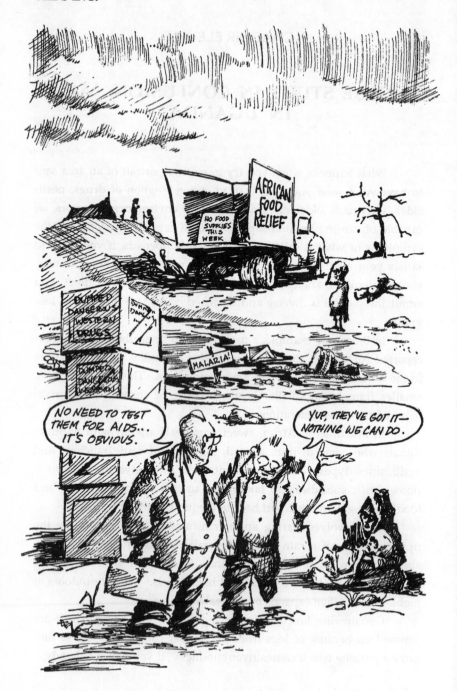

you'll soon be seeing photos of strings of villagers holding hands in chains being led by the only seeing member of the community, a child.

Then there is the human bot-fly. It lays its eggs by first passing them on to mosquitos. When mosquitos land on mammals whose body temperature is close to 98, the survival of the eggs is insured. Cattle, now grazing in large numbers where rain-forests have been torn down, are perfect as incubators.

Increased numbers of bot-flies then drone around and bite people, and the larvae they deposit immediately drill under the skin and excrete a poisonous waste as they grow. Very nasty.

With 2% of Brazil's landowners holding 60% of the arable land in that gigantic country, there is severe dislocation of peasants and severe malnutrition.

The bubonic plague has been found in 41 villages in the northeast. Throughout the country, there are high levels of malaria, TB, polio, leprosy, VD and yellow fever. Malaria is said to produce false-positive results on AIDS blood tests; a fact that may explain some of the hysteria about AIDS.

Then, of course, there are the thousands of backyard pesticide formulators, working with deadly nerve toxins. Who knows what *that* is wreaking?

But as time passes, all this disease and malnutrition comes under the heading, AIDS, a blurring synonym for Disease and All That's Wrong with the Third World.

You will find researchers who make subtle and nice distinctions concerning the three "AIDS" symptoms in the Third World, chronic diarrhea, wasting away (weight-loss), and fever. They will tell you it depends on which organisms are causing the diarrhea, and how fast the wasting is occurring, and so forth, as to whether such a simple thing as malnutrition or traditional illness is really at the root of any given diagnosable AIDS case.

But, as I have pointed out, part of the reason AIDS is being defined so loosely in the first place is that medical care in the Third World is scarce. Labs for good testing are even scarcer. Be as subtle as you want, but under the tremendous pressure of "new disease," doctors will by and large take the grossest aspects of these so-called AIDS symptoms and slap a diagnosis on, bingo. AIDS. That is the way things work.

With all this in mind, let's look at AIDS in Uganda.

This sketch is meant to show that global assumptions about AIDS are not necessarily based on thorough investigation. In Uganda, the questions are: What diseases is that nation really experiencing, and what are the causes? Unlike some analyses, which attempt to establish one root cause, this one attempts to show that diversity is the order of the day, and AIDS is a convenient fiction which fails to consider the complexity of what is really going on.

In the summer of 1987, Uganda received $6 million from the World Health Organization and a number of Western nations, to launch an attack on AIDS. Rated as having the highest number of cases in Africa (1,136), Uganda is supposed to use the money for public education, blood-supply screening, upgrading laboratories for testing, and epidemiological tracking.[1]

There are posters in the capital alerting citizens to the slim disease, which is the local term for wasting away, and is synonymous with AIDS.

According to the Ugandan embassy in Washington, there has been no widespread famine in the country, which is extremely fertile. A drought in a relatively small area of the northeast, in 1980, but no widespread starvation.

A source at the World Bank notes that in the late 1970s and early 80s, and then again in 1985-6, political/military disturbances created pockets in which agricultural production declined and transport of food was impaired. For how long at a stretch? Perhaps a year. How much malnutrition are we talking about? Unanswered.

A *Lancet* article on the 19th of October, 1985, by D. Serwadda et al, announced slim as a new disease in Uganda, and associated it with HIV as the cause. 1982 was pinned as the year of its first appearance, and Serwadda listed its primary symptoms as weight loss and diar-

---

[1] Two sources indicate that the $6 million has yet to be banked in Uganda.

rhea. His study was based on 70 people, most of whom were farmers or other rural residents.

Do not substitute "pastoral" in your mind for "rural," however, at least as far as Serwadda is concerned. He says, "The fact that the disease was first recognized in an exceptionally squalid village suggests that lack of hygiene may be important . . ." But a variety of diseases can flourish in an area of poor sanitation. Were traditional causes of weight-loss and diarrhea checked and eliminated as possibilities? Not known.

Also, what about lack of food in that village?

A followup article in the November 23, 1985 *Lancet* by KH Marquart et al confirms the existence of slim as a disease, and describes two women from Kampala as having its major symptoms – with no protein malnutrition prior to onset. The women had been experiencing, however, vomiting and abdominal pain "for some months," so it is logical to ask if they had become ill from an unknown cause and *then*, because of their symptoms, found it difficult to take in food and so lost weight. No answer.

Meanwhile, under a decade of rule by Idi Amin, the health care system in Uganda collapsed. Doctors left the country. What role this may have played in the appearance of new disease is hard to say. Ugandans, during Amin's rule and later political turmoil, fled into the Sudan. One study indicates that some of the people showing up at the refugee camps there were malnourished.

Another health researcher in Uganda casually mentions weighing children for weight-loss in "busy clinics" with a new time-saving device, which determines if they have "wasting...the most important index of under nutrition." The picture sketched is of patients streaming into clinics who are suffering from lack of food. It seems, in fact, that two parallel tracks of research have been going on in Uganda. One has it that in 1985 a new disease called slim (AIDS), whose primary symptom is weight-loss, appeared; the other track assumes in a down-to-earth manner that wasting is obviously the result of undernutrition.

Now in humans, the animal brucella germ has caused symptoms which overlap pre-AIDS symptoms. In Uganda, since the 1970s, a cattle strain of brucella has, in fact, been causing increasing amounts of human illness. DGK Ndyabattinduka and IH Chu found, in a 1984 study (*Int. Journal Zoonoses*, vol. 11, p. 59) that brucella "is much more widespread than we hitherto considered, particularly in the newly established diary farms...recent data in Uganda indicate that brucellosis is one of the most prevalent zoonoses (diseases of animals that can infect humans) incapacitating labor forces and resulting in tremendous economic loss. A considerable number of cases are found among hospital patients who without lab tests are usually treated (wrongly) for malaria and other chronic illnesses . . ."

The authors list brucellosis symptoms as "malaise, fever, sweating, headache, and muscle pains."

These, in other literature, have been touted as the first signs of Uganda slim disease.

In the August 1986 *Journal of Tropical Medicine and Hygiene,* EH Williams reports on an analysis of 30,129 inpatient admissions, from July 1951 to August 1978, at one Ugandan hospital. Of the six most common causes of admission, diarrhea was the sixth (1041 patients). Was that the "new slim disease" starting in 1951?

Of all the deaths which resulted in those 30,129 patients, 40% were due either to kwashiorkor – which is an immune-deficiency syndrome caused by extreme protein deficiency – or other malnutrition. If you add in a third type of immune-suppression, anemia, you raise the total to 59% of all deaths in those hospital patients.

It is clear in fact that from 1951 on, Ugandans were exhibiting immune suppression in several forms, all of which would give rise to opportunistic infections. The AIDS basic pattern. HIV had nothing to do with any of this.

D. Serwadda's October 1985 *Lancet* paper, discovering slim as a new disease in Uganda, makes this comment, spelling out a typical early slim onset: "In the first six months the patient experiences general malaise and intermittent fevers for which he may treat himself with aspirin, chloroquine, or chloramphenicol. In due course he develops loss of appetite. In the next six months intermittent diarrhea starts. There is gradual weight loss." (KH

Marquart's November 1985 *Lancet* study lists severe vomiting and abdominal pain as slim symptoms, as well.)

Lippincott's 1988 *Drug Factors and Comparisons*, for the drug chloramphenicol, starkly warns: "Serious and fatal blood dyscrasias (aplastic anemia, hypoplastic anemia . . .) occur after chloramphenicol administration."

Reports on use of this antibiotic indicate the occurrence of aplastic anemia has later terminated in leukemia. Side effects include nausea, vomiting, diarrhea, fever. Slim symptoms.

The other drug "early slim" patients were dosing themselves with was chloroquine. Fatalities in children have occurred from its use. Side effects include nausea, vomiting, diarrhea, abdominal cramps, skin pigment changes, raised fungal patches of skin, loss of appetite.

What kind of medical research are we dealing with here?

A new disease is named, slim, after studying patients who have been dosing themselves with very dangerous drugs which yield the same symptoms as the new disease. Chloramphenicol has been routinely dumped by the west in the Third World, even though in the U.S. and Europe, its use is limited because of its danger.

There have been 1600 AIDS cases reported from Uganda since 1983. How many have taken these drugs? Not known.

Finally, Serwadda mentions that, *as early as 1962, aggressive Kaposi's sarcoma* has been seen in Uganda. That further throws doubt on the idea of a global AIDS epidemic, in which aggressive Kaposi's sarcoma was supposedly born simultaneously, in 1980, in San Francisco and Africa.

The understanding of what is being called AIDS in Uganda is very shaky at best. Yet on that foundation, the nation is being held up to the world as the place in Africa where AIDS is most virulent. And the World Health Organization, trying to navigate that continent and win over governments with its plans and programs, is pointing to Uganda as an example of a "cooperative" nation. Last year, Jonathan Mann, WHO AIDS spokesman, held a press conference to announce the $6 million assistance-package. "We all owe a debt to Uganda for its leadership in openly confronting the AIDS problem," he said.

There is more to add to the medical picture in Uganda. More unreported information. My purpose, as I say, is not to reduce disease in that nation to a simple formula – just the opposite. Those who claim to know all about Uganda (or quite probably any Third World country's health situation) are exaggerating wildly.

In my most recent conversation with a Ugandan health official,[2] I discovered that HIV-test facilities in the country are "very poor. The test has a false-positive rate of 17 to 40%," he said. That rate of incorrect result would render it useless as a tool for linking infections with presence of the virus.

There does definitely seem to be a large upsurge in illness in some regions of the country, according to the above source, and the main symptoms are wasting, fever and pain. The illness is lethal, and takes under five years from onset to death. It is different in appearance from any other form of weight-loss he has seen, in that the wasting is quicker. The disease does not seem to be affecting areas in the north where they have had extreme food shortages, although it may be present in the east, another region of food-shortage.

On the whole, food is not a problem in Uganda, the source states. But because of civil strife, government health services have broken down badly. In Kampala, for example, where 20,000 blood transfusions are given every year, blood is not being screened. Infected needles are used. This would mean that scores of *various* microbes would be passed directly into recipients' bloodstreams, causing all sorts of unspecified health problems.

In Uganda, infant mortality, for all reasons, has climbed considerably, to over 120 deaths per thousand live births. The official had no knowledge of how many reported AIDS cases or current unreported cases of wasting are among children. This seems to be a difficult figure to come by. It is generally held that in Africa, reported AIDS among children is at a higher ratio than in the West.

---

[2] All health people I spoke with about Uganda refused to go on the record. Reason? Unclear. In some cases, it may have been because being diagnosed with AIDS in Uganda seems to be a disgrace. Therefore, officials prefer to keep silent altogether about the subject.

This official said chloramphenicol was not available in areas where the wasting disease is occurring.

No post-mortems are being done on victims of any disease in Uganda. Therefore, there is no hard knowledge from that useful avenue on what diseases and conditions are killing people.

If there is a new disease in Uganda, it has not been definitively diagnosed. If it is a more virulent version of an old disease, that has not been discovered either.

Question marks.

It is not easy to find out which pesticides have been used in Uganda. But a 1985 report,[3] not widely distributed, indicates that, at least since 1970, "malpractices have occurred. Numerous agricultural pesticides of unknown purity, without labels and largely of doubtful effectiveness, found their way to the farmers." The report goes on to note that no laws exist in Uganda to regulate safety procedures in handling, storing, using, or protecting against pesticides and their residues.

Beginning in 1985, the U.S.-banned pesticide dieldrin has definitely been reported in Uganda. An organochlorine, it is a powerful nerve toxin whose effects are cumulative; so the immediate warning of a strong adverse physical reaction does not necessarily exist for users. Dieldrin creeps up the food chain as well.

A 1977 FDA report, "Pesticides in Imported Coffee Beans," indicated that the one tested sample of beans from Uganda was contaminated by pesticides. No chemical contaminant was named, but the general list of those found in bean samples from 22 countries included DDT, Dieldrin, malathion, and Lindane, all highly toxic compounds.

Illness to workers in pesticide plants abroad and to farm workers handling toxins is vastly underreported. In many Third World nations, this sort of illness could be, and probably is, reported under other names, including AIDS.

---

[3] "Pesticide Management in East and Southern Africa," published in 1985 by the US Agency for International Development, presented at the proceedings of a workshop held in Nairobi, 10-15 Mar. 1985; edited and compiled by Janice Jensen, Ann Stroud, and Joy Mukanyange.

Another report on Uganda comes from a Western scientist who spent part of the summer of 1987 there. He stated that there are at least three diseases which are severe in the country, and none of them is being widely discussed. One is malaria, on the rise, another is a venereal infection called ulcerating chancroid, "which has been reported in perhaps one out of 10 adults," the scientists told me. "This could mean one out of three sexually active adults have that infection," he said.

The third disease is tick-borne relapsing fever, which produces off and on undulating fevers. It is prevalent along a 20-mile road outside Kampala, a road which used to be well kept and was easy to travel. Now, however, after years of war, it can take eight hours in a four-wheel vehicle to cover those 20 miles. That means lots of stops, and that means exposure to the ticks.

AIDS, the scientist told me, has come to be a label which makes a pariah out of a person in Uganda. Therefore, if people with this tick fever are misdiagnosed as having AIDS, they are put out from their homes, cut off from their families, refused food and any available medication – which surely would worsen their illness.

No one is testing pigs for swine fever in Uganda, but some pigs still roam freely in areas where people have been diagnosed with AIDS. Swine fever has been known to produce wasting-away in pigs, and some scientists report it can infect humans.

Sanitation facilities in the country are, the scientist reported, very poor. Perhaps a quarter of the people have latrines. This situation, of course, creates a breeding ground for all sorts of disease.

There are very few medical drugs available in the country. The doctors, this scientist reports, who are part of the socialized medical system, are paid about $12 a month in salary. With $30 as the bare minumum for survival, doctors may sell drugs they receive on the black market, then give smaller amounts to patients and stretch out the available supplies. In 1967, doctors were treating VD in the country with small doses of penicillin. The symptoms would recede, although the disease was probably not wiped out, and when symptoms surfaced later, they were resistant to penicillin.

This visiting scientist saw no pesticide plants or pesticide use, but wasn't looking for that sort of thing. However, he did mention that a lake in the Rakai district, where AIDS has been diagnosed, was not producing fish anymore and no one seemed to know why.

Malnutrition was not a problem in the country, the scientist reported. Land is very fertile, and crops almost grow by themselves.

He felt that some illness was being misdiagnosed as AIDS, and, at the same time, some new disease, probably contagious, was also killing people. Origin unknown, but possibly tick-borne. Its symptoms were vomiting, diarrhea, and weight-loss. It didn't seem to be tick-borne relapsing fever.

Another scientist, Jane Teas, sent a letter to Senator Ted Kennedy after returning from a 1985 trip to Uganda. It was reprinted in the September 30, 1985, *New York Native,* and introduced the subject of African Swine Fever in Uganda for the first time. Here is a brief excerpt from Teas' letter:

"(My trip to Uganda led to) extensive inquiries; I found that there was an ongoing epidemic of African Swine Fever Virus, as well as a civil war in Uganda. Since Uganda might suffer economically if they formally diagnosed the disease in pigs, no one has officially tested the pigs for African Swine Fever Virus. When I was in Uganda, in May 1984, there were thought to have been six cases of AIDS in Kampala. Now, just over a year later, there are more than 60 cases in one hospital alone. The pigs in Kampala, as elsewhere in Uganda, roam freely in people's gardens, and are not restricted to pig farms."[4]

The bottom line on all these health reports about Uganda is that no one has the bottom line on what is killing people in that country. Those who say they do, and I have talked to some, are molding a characterization that fits their ideas about AIDS. Several of these people, of course, claim special prescience, in an almost religious way. Well, there are many possible payoffs in asserting there is

---

[4] African Swine Fever has reportedly been found in the blood of some AIDS patients.

one cause for one global epidemic that encompasses virtually all human immunosuppression.

If the truth is less easy to come by, that has never stopped people determined to sell a theory. Unfortunately for them, AIDS is blatantly a hodge-podge of symptoms which can be produced from many quarters. It is also a very familiar pattern: immune-suppression permitting outbreaks of opportunistic infections. Hundreds of initiating factors can give rise to that precise pattern.

CHAPTER TWELVE

DOES THE HIV VIRUS CAUSE DISEASE?

If the AIDS research establishment has a leg to stand on, it is accomplished by claiming that the HIV virus actually causes the collapse of the human immune system; that HIV therefore paves the way for all the symptoms and diseases and infections that are considered AIDS-associated.

Of course, top AIDS researchers believe HIV does *exactly* these things, and so the question is: How do they prove it? Because it must not be forgotten, the burden of proof was and is on those who claim HIV causes disease.

Traditionally, in order to establish that a germ causes a condition, medical researchers invoke what are called Koch's postulates.

These postulates describe a formula: From people with a given disease, remove the same germ in every case; then inject this germ into animals and in every case bring about all the symptoms of the disease.

Having accomplished this, one says that germ A causes disease B.

With HIV, this has not been done. First, depending on which study you read, you find HIV itself has been isolated in roughly 50-80% of those people diagnosed with full-blown AIDS. Second, about a hundred chimps in the U.S., held in sterile isolation chambers, have been injected with high volumes of HIV. Two chimps immediately developed infected lymph glands; this condition lasted for thirty weeks and then returned to normal. In those two chimps, no new symptoms then appeared. In all the other chimps, no AIDS-like symptoms developed at all.

It has been over four years since at least some of these 100 chimps have been injected with HIV.

83

So on the basis of Koch's postulates, there are no grounds for positively asserting that HIV causes AIDS.

Several researchers claim that in the past some other disease-germs have been discovered without fulfilling Koch's postulates; and that HIV, belonging to a special class called retroviruses, needs to be judged by different criteria than the postulates. But these criteria have not been debated or made clear in published papers. They have only been bandied about.

HIV advocates have also invoked what is called transfusion-AIDS. The thinking goes this way. Healthy people with no background of "high-risk" activity, when transfused with blood containing HIV, have developed full-blown AIDS. Therefore, the obvious cause was HIV, and this proves HIV causes AIDS.

On the surface, it seems like sound reasoning. However, looking over available statistics on people who get transfusions, a different picture emerges.

Calculating from figures supplied by the American Association of Blood Banks, since 1978 about 29 million Americans have received blood transfusions. In most of these transfusions, more than one donor supplied the various pints injected, so there was ample opportunity to receive HIV in the bloodstream. The average size of a transfusion is 3.5 pints.

As of February 1988, the CDC reports a total of 1466 transfusion AIDS in the US (since AIDS was first reported). This means that about .00005 of those who have received transfusions in the last ten years have been diagnosed with AIDS. That's 5/hundred thousandths of one percent.

On that basis, could you possibly infer that HIV is the cause of something called AIDS? Obviously not. One could argue that these statistics don't absolutely *rule out* HIV as a sometime cause of human disease, but this is not the question. Many researchers who attribute AIDS to HIV state, *as proof*, blood-transfusion AIDS. The burden of proof is on them. Their scenario doesn't hold up in this area.

In addition, several transfusion-AIDS enthusiasts say that, since mass-screening of hospital blood-reserves for HIV began, transfusion-AIDS has virtually been eliminated; therefore the culprit

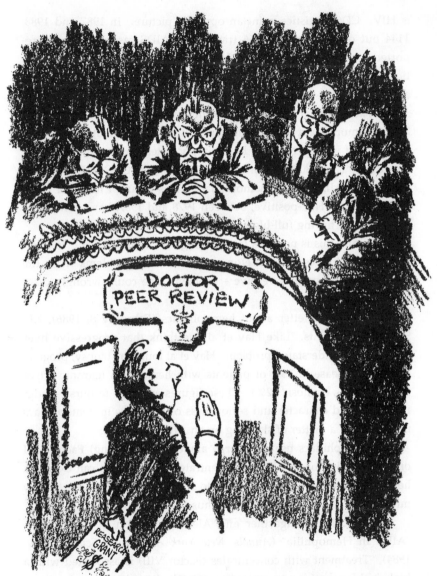

"I DO SOLEMNLY SWEAR THAT *HIV* IS THE SOLE CAUSE OF *AIDS*, AND I WILL UPHOLD *HIV'S* RIGHT TO BE THE ONE AND ONLY..."

is HIV. CDC statistics paint an opposite picture. In 1987 and 1988, 1144 out of the total of 1466 transfusion-AIDS cases have been reported. In other words, since HIV has been filtered out of the national blood supply, reported transfusion-AIDS has risen considerably.

The National Hemophilia Foundation reports there are about 20,000 hemophiliacs of different types in the United States. Slippery estimates of what percentage have simply tested positive for HIV vary between 50% and 80%. As of January 11, 1987, the CDC reports 543 total cases of AIDS among hemophiliacs. This means 4 to 5% of those *estimated* to be HIV-positive, between 1978 and 1987, have gone to be diagnosed as having full-blown AIDS.

Again, this is no basis for claiming HIV causes AIDS.[1] In addition, hemophiliacs can develop other immune problems from the many transfusions they receive – problems one could wrongly disgnose as AIDS.

In a *Lancet* letter about hemophiliacs (February 8, 1986), KL. Schimpf comments, "Like Hay et al, we think that progressive liver disease is an understated problem. Hay et al found by biopsy, progressive liver disease in 38% of patients with hemophilia (chronic active hepatitis 26%, cirrhosis 12%). These figures are close to ours." Judging the varied character and seriousness of problems in hemophiliacs is not simply a matter of slapping on an AIDS diagnosis.

Hemophiliacs use very large amounts of (clotting) Factor VIII on a continuing basis. These concentrates from plasma can expose a hemophiliac to the blood of 100,000 to 300,000 donors per year. *Many* microbial toxins and chemicals can thus be passed on.

As authors Hilgartner and Aledort mention in their paper, "AIDS in Hemophilia" (*Annals, New York Academy of Science*, Nov. 1984), "Treatment with concentrates (Factor VIII) is associated with a high incidence of cytomegalovirus (CMV), hepatitis B, and non-A-non-B hepatitis." Immune disorders found in hemophiliacs include hemolytic anemia and ITP, an autoimmune blood platelet problem.

---

[1] As with transfusion-recipients in general, counting the raw numbers of transfusions received by hemophiliacs would yield a similar microscopic percentage of those eventually diagnosed with AIDS.

These non-viral conditions can result in the outbreak of opportunistic infections, and in this pattern they are virtually indistinguishable from AIDS.

In the discussion following the Hilgartner and Aledort paper, which was initially presented at an AIDS symposium, a questioner said, "The hemophiliac population in Germany and Central Europe is about one-third of the same population of the United States. These patients are treated with similar or rather slightly higher doses of concentrates. They are comparable . . . and there was not a single case of AIDS reported."

Hilgartner replied, "That, I think, is one of the most important facts that we have heard. In a population treated with even larger amounts of concentrate than we have used in the United States for a period of three to five years, there is as yet no indication of AIDS. If there had been a contaminated lot or if there had been a virus or transmissible agent, one would certainly have thought that at least one case would have appeared at the present time in those German hemophiliacs."

One can certainly speculate on this strange fact, but regardless, invoking hemophilia to prove HIV causes AIDS just isn't going to work.

What would be the likelihood of scientists reversing their field if HIV were somehow discredited? Realistically, about zero. In this regard, biologist Peter Duesberg had a few interesting things to say to reporter Celia Farber for *Spin* magazine (January 1988):

"Scientists researching AIDS are much less inclined to ask scrutinizing questions about the etiology (cause) of AIDS when they have invested huge sums of money in companies that make money on the hypothesis that HIV is the AIDS virus. William Haseltine and Max Essex, for example, who are two of the top five AIDS researchers in the country, have millions in stocks in a company they founded that has developed and will sell AIDS kits that test for HIV. How could they be objective? Gallo stands to make a lot of money from patent rights on the virus. His entire reputation depends on this virus. If HIV is not the cause of AIDS, there's nothing left for Gallo."

Farber found researchers Hazeltine and Essex upset by Duesberg's remarks, but she added that Hazeltine "confirms his and Essex's business arrangement with Cambridge Bio-Science, a company that sells HIV testing kits."

A gay man from Ohio told me that, in the late 1970s, he and a number of friends had vacationed in New York, San Francisco, and Los Angeles, the three cities where an overwhelming percentage of AIDS among gay men has been diagnosed.

"We all went to the bathhouses, we returned home to our cities. These cities never developed anywhere near the percentage of AIDS among us as in, say, San Francisco."

This is true.

With gay men from all over the U.S. taking vacation trips to San Francisco, New York, and LA, a transmissible AIDS-causing HIV virus would have been transported back to Des Moines, Atlanta, Sandusky, Salt Lake City, and many other cities and towns across America. AIDS would, by now, be showing a very wide distribution across the U.S., among gays.

This has not happened, according to reports.

The conclusion? Perhaps that a vacation is not long enough to absorb the necessary quantity of drugs which, along with STDs, actually comprise much of the immunosuppressive effect called AIDS.

On the international scene, no one has been able to explain the odd distribution of reported AIDS cases – assuming a virus is doing the job. Why do we have a reported preponderance of heterosexual Africans and homosexual Americans with AIDS; why don't we have many more cases in Europe, since that continent's connections with Africa are traditionally so much stronger than America's? Ordinarily, one would think, if AIDS started in Africa, it would gain a very strong foothold there, lots of reported cases would show up, and *then* it would appear in America and Europe, and begin to fan out slowly. It wouldn't erupt in America simultaneously, and build up to 40,000 cases here.

Meanwhile, in the laboratory, researchers have said that HIV is the likely cause of AIDS because it kills T-cells in petri dishes At the time this claim was made, AIDS was considered to be a damager of T-cells in the human body. Now, some researchers have shifted their position and said that the HIV virus actually attacks the immune-cells called the macrophages, instead.

Regardless, many things, chemical and microbial, can kill human cells in petri dishes. In dishes, there is no immune-response at work; the normal processes of the human body are not functioning. This fact is known to every high-school biology student.

In a later chapter, I interview a molecular biologist on the subject of HIV. One of the vital points he makes concerns the transmissibility of HIV. There is no question that it can be passed from one person to another. This is true of many microbes, none of which cause us harm. There is no reason to assume that because a germ moves from person to person it causes disease.

Going around the world warning of imminent disaster based on the fact that people test positive for the HIV virus...this is a successful strategy to make people think we have a transmitted HIV plague on our hands, but it is not science or anything bordering on it.

It is also very easy to move into a country where certain diseases crop up now and then. Take a Third World country where, every decade or so, they have an epidemic of cholera. But instead of treating the latest horrible outbreak in the usual way (for example, by improving sanitation), researchers on the scene say, "Cholera is an opportunistic infection of AIDS. The reason it is happening is the prior immune-damage in the bodies of these citizens. Damage caused by HIV. As proof, we will test some of these people."

They do, and lo and behold, they find antibodies to the HIV virus. Now they say, "You see? HIV. What did we tell you? Aha. AIDS."

Robert Gallo and Flossie Wong-Staal (*Nature,* 3 October, 1985) offered five reasons for HIV being the cause of AIDS.

1) CDC studies on hemophiliacs who receive clotting Factor VIII are then diagnosed with AIDS.

2) In AIDS patients, there are apparent defects in immune T-cell populations, and HIV has been found to destroy T-cells in vitro.

3) A virus similar to HIV, feline leukemia virus, is known to cause a similar disease to AIDS.

4) HTLV-I and HTLV-II, similar to HIV, have shown the capacity to induce immune suppression in vitro.

5) AIDS started in Africa and Haiti, both known to be endemic for the HTLV-I and II viruses.

In retrospect, the replies to this "evidence" are quite obvious.

1) The percentage of hemophiliacs who are diagnosed with AIDS is tiny. At any rate, some hemophiliacs already suffer from immune-deficiency indistinguishable from AIDS.

2) Many germs and chemicals (and malnutrition) can cause defects in immune T-cell populations, and destruction of T-cells in a petri dish is not proof that HIV does anything in the body.

3) Feline leukemia virus is normally present in 70% of cats. It has not been shown to cause leukemia.

4) HTLV-I and HTLV-II are not now thought to be part of the family to which HIV belongs. So the comparison is irrelevant.

5) Same objection as #4. Also, the prediction of huge numbers of AIDS cases in Haiti by now has not, from reports, panned out. In 1985, roughly 360,000 Haitians were said to be on the road to AIDS because they were, by statistical projection, positive for the HIV virus. In 1988, we have 920 reported cases of AIDS in Haiti.[2] Similarly, in Africa, fast surveys in Kenya and Uganda brought predictions of millions of AIDS cases. Later, more sober analysis of blood-test results there indicated overwhelming numbers of *falsely* positive HIV tests.[3]

There is a myth that "everyone knows HIV causes AIDS." Like other myths, when you begin to talk to people, you find the myth has cracks, and people are often afraid to voice their real opinions. I found this to be so when I spoke with university researchers. It also appears to be true within the White House itself, and signals a probable conflict over this issue at high policy levels.

Senior White House policy analyst Jim Warner first came to public attention in a November article in the *New York Native*. In the story, "The White House Calls the Native About Aids," publisher

---

[2] See Curran et al, *Science*, v. 229, p. 1352, 1985; Tinker, *Issues in Science and Technology*, no. 4, p. 43, 1988.

[3] Schneider et al, "Seroepidemiology of HIV in Africa," *British Medical Journal*, Sept. 27, 1986.

Chuck Ortleb wrote: "Warner told me that the White House could be seen as divided into two groups on the issue of AIDS. One group, which he said is in the minority, wants to adopt an 'Auschwitz model' by quarantining all those infected with 'the virus.' 'The other group,' [Warner] said, 'is incompetent.'" Later, Warner told me he wasn't suggesting there was a White House group which was favoring "an Auschwitz model," but that some high-risk groups might *think* that was so. The following interview ran in the *LA Weekly* on December 18, 1987.

WEEKLY: *Has anyone at the White House spoken to you about the* Native *article and what you said in it?*
WARNER: I don't think anyone here knows there was an article in that paper.

The government really hasn't fulfilled its role in providing good information [on AIDS]. We just may not know enough. With AIDS, we're dealing with a syndrome, not a disease. We may see a patient who has a genetic defect that's causing his immune deficiency [instead of HIV being the causative agent]. I'm not satisfied we know all we think we do, by any means.
WEEKLY: *Is your research on AIDS part of your policy work? Do you make recommendations based on what you find out? Or is it just that you're absorbed in discovering what's going on with AIDS?*
WARNER: More of the latter than the former. I was asked to look into an *Atlantic* magazine article about insects and AIDS, and that's how it started. I decided I wanted to put together a set of questions concerning the HIV virus, so that the answers would suggest its role in AIDS. I would then draft a paper and give it to the people who asked me to look into the subject.
WEEKLY: *Do people at the White House get a chance to talk to scientists over at the National Institutes of Health? I mean really talk with them, find out what they're doing, how they're thinking?*
WARNER: There is not much communication [between people at the White House and the scientists at NIH]. I'm probably the only person here who has much interest in it. This year I determined that the [White House] working group on AIDS wasn't adequate.

WEEKLY: *Several university scientists I've spoken with have – off the record – criticized what they call "HIV dogma." They feel if they speak out against the rush to judgment for HIV as the cause of AIDS they may lose money. Grants begin with the assumption that HIV has been proven as the agent of the disease.*

WARNER: I'm of a mind that if no other lessons should be required of any university science curriculum, there should be a good survey course in philosophy and a grounding in logic. I'm appalled at the conceit and arrogance [of certain scientists].

WEEKLY: *There has never been a performanace-evaluation on the results of the NIH. NIH has balked at the idea of evaluating the worth of all their medical research over the last 20 years.*

WARNER: That's a very good idea. I'm going to see what I can do about that.

WEEKLY: *The Native article mentioned that you spoke with Dr. Lo, an Army researcher on AIDS. He has his own theory about the disease, that it's caused by a different virus. According to the Native, you had a problem getting through to him. Did they really tell you you'd have to get an okay from the Surgeon General just to talk to Lo?*

WARNER: Yes. You know, although it is an honor to work at the White House, I'm not impressed that being here makes me special. But I pulled rank, and they put me through to Dr. Lo.

WEEKLY: *Suppose proof emerged that HIV is not the AIDS virus. How difficult would it be to alter the course of research?*

WARNER: It's very difficult to change people's minds. It's not impossible, but there is a head of steam built up.

WEEKLY: *What do you do if a government agency, as a whole, has been derelict?*

WARNER: It may end up as a brawl. I'd sort of like to finesse that, though, I'd like to avoid a public brawl. It eats up time. It's difficult when scientists are not open to discussing scientific issues.

WEEKLY: *Robert Gallo, Max Essex, people like that, were the field commanders on the NIH war on cancer in the 70's. They lost that war. So why are they in charge of AIDS research now? It seems odd that we don't have other people running the show.*

WARNER: If ever I've been tempted to believe in socialism, science has disabused me of that. These guys [at NIH] assume that it's their show. They just assume it.

WEEKLY: *Peter Duesberg, a distinguished molecular biologist at Berkeley, has said that HIV does not cause AIDS. Have you asked people at NIH what they think, specifically, of his arguments?*

WARNER: Yes. I've been told that Peter Duesberg's refutation of HIV has been discounted by the scientific community. I was given no explanation as to why. I was very offended. No evidence was presented to me. Just that Duesberg had been 'discounted.' That's absurd. It's not a scientific response to dismiss Duesberg as a crank.

WEEKLY: *The definition of AIDS has become so broad it's even stretching the idea of what a syndrome is, never mind a singular disease.*

WARNER: A syndrome is a means of trying to understand how symptoms could be linked together. But if you do this in an atmosphere of hysteria, there is no limit to what you can attribute to a syndrome.

WEEKLY: *The definition of AIDS in Africa is now becoming synonymous with starvation. They're saying the three major symptoms are chronic diarrhea, fever, and wasting-away. Weight-loss. It certainly makes a perfect smokescreen for the aspect of hunger which is political – just call it AIDS.*

WARNER: I had not considered that. There is a program to make Africa self-sufficient by the year 2000. This could certainly hinder that activity.

You know, I was a prisoner of war in Vietnam. I experienced weight-loss of eighty pounds. And when I came home, I was suffering from a form of dysentery that you could call opportunistic. A number of us were. We didn't have AIDS.

In November of 1987, I found out that the journal *Bio/Technology*, was going to hold a roundtable workshop in which

HIV would be addressed. Peter Duesberg and about a dozen other researchers would attend. The purpose of the roundtable would be to formulate experiments which, once and for all, would show HIV's role or non-role in AIDS.

I told Jim Warner about the proposed roundtable, and suggested he contact the magazine and sit in on the sessions. He did call, and to everyone's surprise, suggested that the roundtable be held in his office at the White House.

For the next month, it was on again, off again. There were obviously pressures within the White House against sanctioning such a meeting. About a month before the scheduled January 19th date, stories about it began appearing in several newspapers.

For a brief time, it looked like the White House's Office of Policy Development was not going to host it, but the Office of Science and Technology Policy was. Then the whole thing fell apart.

The *New York Post,* on January 7th, 1988, ran a story on Duesberg. The next day, the paper did a followup, headlined: U.S. AXES DEBATE ON TRUE CAUSE OF AIDS. After indicating that the White House meeting was canceled, medicine-science editor, Joe Nicholson, relayed a few surprising quotes from Gary Bauer, head of Reagan's Office of Policy Development, and Jim Warner's boss:

"People like Dr. Duesberg need to continue to have access to research funds so that if we are heading in the wrong direction, that can be proved."

Bauer then said he didn't want the White House to sponsor the meeting because it would impart a political tone to a scientific event.

"I hope they have the debate elsewhere," he said. "I've sort of bristled at the finality with which some have made statements about AIDS and how it is transmitted. When findings run counter to the accepted wisdom, there is a tendency to muzzle or ignore rather than have an open debate."

The average researcher will tell you that there is an extraordinary correlation which proves beyond a shadow of a doubt that HIV causes AIDS: One new disease-condition has sprung up simultaneously around the globe; called AIDS, it is everywhere accompanied by the presence of a virus, HIV, which is also new; this correlation of new disease and new virus cannot be a casual thing without meaning; HIV must actually cause AIDS.

This is a compelling image for researchers, this correlation, and it is why, at bottom, they are so sure that HIV causes AIDS.

But the truth is, a new disease-condition has not demonstrably sprung up all over the world.[4] Hundreds of causes for immune-system collapse and ensuing infection, the so-called AIDS pattern, already exist. There is nothing magical about the ideas of AIDS. It is merely immune-collapse followed by opportunistic infection.

What is actually correlated with "new disease" around the world is positive HIV blood tests.[5] These tests do not detect the virus, but the response of the immune system to a contact with the virus. That response is measured by the presence of immune-troops called antibodies. Normally, antibodies are thought to signal a successfully mounted effort against the intrusion of a germ. Exceptions have certainly been reported, in which antibodies did not ward off illness. However, to assume *across the board* that the generation of antibodies to one virus, HIV, in all cases, signifies *future death* as a result of that virus is to turn around established understanding.

If that is the new analysis, it must be accompanied by extensive proof that a blood test for HIV which shows antibodies will definitely mean later disease. This proof has not been offered. The largest attempt is being made, at the San Francisco City Clinic, where two specialized groups of men are being tracked, to see how many of them eventually are diagnosed with full-blown AIDS years after being labeled positive for HIV on blood tests.

Unfortunately, these groups are very specialized, and it would be foolish to imagine that information about the general population can be extracted from them. One large group, for example, consists of men who showed up at STD clinics in San Francisco in the late 1970s. Many of these men were certainly already immune-compromised, as a result of successive incidents of STDs and massive antibiotic usage.

---

4 See Chapter 13, *Pneumocystis*.

5 See Chapter 31, which analyzes the unreliability of HIV blood tests.

The other group being studied are gay men who volunteered for the early Hepatitis B vaccine trials in 1980.

A large percentage of the men in the San Francisco study would fall under the category of "high-risk" for AIDS, by the CDC guidelines. The idea that data from them could be extrapolated to people whose lives, habits, exposures to chemicals are totally different is flawed.

Furthermore, the San Francisco study is not complete, and full disclosure of their data, their methods of collection, their protocols has not been offered. Nevertheless, reporters and scientists and MDs have jumped the gun and made indisputable fact out of this study.

In an effort to defend a viral AIDS scenario, in which AIDS has mainly been confined to IV drug users and male homosexuals in the US, researchers have attempted to discover odd routes of viral transmission which occur only in those groups: Anal sex among gays, which because of bleeding leads to semen-blood transmission; and sharing of needles among junkies.

This effort is misguided for several reasons.

No virus selects lopsidedly the cultural groups it will reside in. (By now, ample opportunity has been created for HIV to move out of gays and IV drug users into the general population, and yet this has not happened.)

If HIV were causing a single disease-entity called AIDS, two circumstances in America would have conspired to send AIDS widely beyond the current risk-groups. There existed in New York, in the 1970s, bisexual swing clubs. These active establishments, by eyewitness account, played host to every crossover sex act imaginable and a consequent exchange of bodily fluids among men and women. A perfect situation for viral spread into the hetero community. It didn't happen.

In fact, today out of the 55,000 reported AIDS cases in the US, 91% are men, and 9% are women. That is not the reflection of any known virus at work. Such preference is unheard of.

During the 1970s, as already mentioned, gay men from cities and towns all over America visited and vacationed in San Francisco, New York, and LA, the centers of diagnosed AIDS cases in the US.

They visited gay bathhouses and had sex. Carrying home with them the HIV virus, they would have spread AIDS into many, many towns and cities of the US. This did not occur, according to all available reports.

Among IV drug users, one of the only studies that has tried to show a link between a positive HIV test and the sharing of needles has failed. Comparing a white and a black group of IV drug users, it was found that the group which shared *more* needles tested positive for HIV *less* frequently.

Likewise for anal intercourse, the attempt to show that this "homosexual sex" explains the preference of HIV for gays overlooks the following:

1. Heterosexuals have been practicing anal sex for centuries.

2. Semen to blood transmission, which has been attributed to anal sex as the reason HIV spreads, is also a fact in hetero vaginal sex. Any urban gynecologist will tell you that a certain small percentage of his hetero male and female patients come in with penile and vaginal abrasions. That would also give blood transmission.

Nevertheless, investigators have been fixated on investigating high-risk groups with the theory already firmly in mind that HIV causes AIDS. Based on this, they look for these "idiosyncratic" ways the virus has been transmitted within these groups, ways which wouldn't occur in the general public. They have failed.

Trying to confirm that HIV causes AIDS by showing it spreads in culturally prejudiced fashion, through odd routes, in very limited fashion, is absurd.

If HIV has not been proven to cause AIDS, the next obvious question is, Is AIDS contagious? The answer to that is: If HIV has not been shown to be the link that ties together the 30-odd infections and diseases said to be AIDS related, then what AIDS are you talking about in the first place?

If HIV is not locked in as disease-agent, then all the so-called opportunistic infections of AIDS drift apart, no longer a syndrome.

There are two opportunistic diseases which have been attributed to AIDS, the two most prominent, which are cited to indicate that AIDS is a single root. These two diseases are pneumocystis pneumonia and Kaposi's sarcoma. Researchers have analyzed them in such a way that they appear to give credence to the existence of something called AIDS. But that analysis is superficial and wrong.

The next two chapters take up pneumocystis and Kaposi.

It isn't really surprising that the AIDS research establishment in America is arrogant, when you look at the thesis about AIDS which they have built. Their arrogance is hiding an extremely weak brand of science, protecting it against calm scrutiny.

Try this analogy. A famous researcher, backed up by ample funds and PR people, announces that a gigantic meteor is heading for Earth, and will destroy it. The meteor is invisible, but we know its path because there are very slight variations which have been developing in the orbits of heavenly bodies along a certain route. Caused, it is argued, by the gravity exerted by the meteor.

The meteor will arrive sometime in the next 10-100 years. We can't be sure of the time, because its velocity is not uniform. Why is the velocity erratic? Answer unknown.

Now it is the job of the scientific community to advance the frontiers of technology so that we can somehow divert this meteor and survive as a species.

In this atmosphere of hysteria, other skeptical scientists undertake to check this Earth-collision hypothesis, to see if it really stands up to investigation. How would they check it? That is the question.

Well, it turns out that this is virtually impossible, because the theory has been formed in such an elastic way that it can be stretched in various ways to cover unexpected changes in facts. If Earth doesn't explode in ten years, for example, it's easy to say, 'Oh, we miscalculated the velocity of the meteor. That meteor is tricky. What a bastard. Keeps changing speed. But wait. In another ten or fifty years it'll collide with Earth and blow us all up."

Aside from this ridiculous elasticity, there turns out to be another factor which discredits this meteor theory. There are *already* slight changes in orbits of heavenly bodies in the path of the supposed, invisible meteor. These changes have been taking place for the last billion years, and there are five or six good reasons why, which we already understand. In fact, slight variations in orbits of heavenly bodies take place all over the universe, not just "in the route of the meteor."

Therefore, imagining a meteor was coming toward us *because* these bodies were fluctuating slightly in their ordinary orbits was an unwarranted assumption.

Conclusion? The meteor theory, as concocted, from the existence of the meteor itself to its time of supposed impact, is so vaporous *that it can't be checked.* It's a terrifying proposal but it's gobbledegook.

In exactly the same way, the "theory" of AIDS as proposed, once the smokescreen clears away, is absurd. If we say, "The 500,000 cases of full-blown AIDS in Central Africa haven't developed as you predicted they would," researchers blithely reply, "Wait. It wasn't three years. It was twelve. It'll happen in the year 2000." And if in 2000 nothing happens that just means the date was off again. Try 2020.

Furthermore, since AIDS is nothing more than a label for a condition which already existed prior to the "discovery" of AIDS–namely immune-suppression and resultant infection–the whole theory collapses before it can be formulated. We've known about fifteen or twenty medical reasons and hundreds of environmental causes for immune-deficiency, and we've known about them for decades. Nothing new there. Nothing unique.

So when some people say in despair, "Nobody really knows what's causing AIDS," that's misleading. The truth is, AIDS as formulated can't be checked out one way or another. Of course, as I pointed out in the first chapter, you can always use the real fact that people are dying to shout down any opposition to the scenario called AIDS. But the scenario, when you take it apart, is not only scientifically absurd, it also keeps help for dying and ill people, true help, from taking place. It keeps prevention from taking place. So the AIDS theory isn't just stupid, it's vicious.

As you'll see in later chapters, the definitions of AIDS which are being used around the world will provide, by poaching on the territories of much older diseases, the necessary case statistics to make it seem that we have a global epidemic (from a single viral cause) on our hands. So the AIDS theory, by essentially co-opting other diseases and environmentally caused conditions under its fictional umbrella, will make it seem as if all the terror being generated is justified.

CHAPTER THIRTEEN

PNEUMOCYSTIS, THE PRIMARY AIDS SYMPTOM

If HIV rests in suspended animation, unproven as the cause of disease, what then?

First, it is now foolish to talk about a single entity called AIDS. The only thing that seemed to tie together the many diverse infections and diseases under that title was the HIV virus.

Putting aside HIV, it is much more probable that what is being called AIDS, in most cases, is the far end of an arc of immunosuppression, which takes some time to build up in a person.

From various factors, the immunosuppression gains in influence, and then, long after the person should have reversed his habits, or should have been fed, or should have been taken from a field where he was working in the presence of pesticides, etc., he becomes really sick, and *then* maybe he sees a doctor.

The doctor looks at his opportunistic infections, clucks, pronounces AIDS, and everyone is fearful because the condition has been touted as invariably fatal. Well, at this point in the arc, the chances have naturally increased that it will be irreversible.

But this is flim-flam, since what is defined as AIDS is precisely the end of the arc of immunosuppression. All attention is focused there. It is named AIDS, it is packaged, and what is concealed is the long approach that led to this moment. Prevention and reversal would have been much easier during that earlier period.

Before dissecting the current definitions of AIDS and seeing how they operate in a destructive way, there are one or two myths to take care of.

The first is pneumocystis carinii pneumonia, the primary so-called AIDS symptom. About 32,000 cases of AIDS, since the beginning, have been reported to the CDC because of that symptom, out of a rough total of 55,000 AIDS cases.

The myth of pneumocystis is that it was extremely rare before AIDS, that it was almost unknown, in fact. The other myth is that if two people have pneumocystis, they both developed it from the same cause. That is preposterous.

In 1980-1, the first five cases of gay men with pneumocystis were reported to the CDC from Los Angeles. The CDC report on these cases, and a commentary, are the subject of a later appendix. For now, it's sufficient to say that the examining doctors assumed these five men had developed pneumocystis for the same reason, when a search of the literature on the disease would have shown that that is a very shaky assumption.

Promoting pneumocystis as very rare and coming from *one* unknown cause did a great deal to convince people that we had a new disease on our hands: AIDS. A more thorough understanding about pneumocystis would have shown that there was less to fear, more that could be done in the way of prevention.

The pneumocystis protozoa is found in 70-85% of healthy people. It causes no harm. It is one of those germs which establishes an easy relationship with the host. However, when immunosuppression becomes severe enough, it can come to the fore, center in the lungs, and cause virulent disease.

This is the starting point for understanding pneumocystis.

1980 in a loose way marks the beginning of health-agency awareness about AIDS, but 1977-8 is usually the more precise period for dividing pre-AIDS and post-AIDS time.

In 1977, doctors also began routinely performing a new method for detecting pneumocystis pneumonia at the Eugene Talmadge Memorial Hospital in Georgia. It's called percutaneous lung aspirate. From January 1955 to July 1977, the hospital had observed seven cases of pneumocystis. But from July 1977 to December 1979, "nine episodes occurred in seven patients."[1]

---

[1] December 1980 *Southern Medical Journal*, Frederick Cox et al, "Pneumocystis Recognition in Hospitals: Outbreaks or Improved Recognition."

Although the study does not prove higher incidence of pneumocystis was due to a better method of detection, it does give pause for thought.

Various studies indicate that the pneumocystis organism causes no harm until some immuno-adversity arises: often immunosuppressive drug therapy or an organ transplant. A host of other immunosuppressive factors can lead to pneumocystis pneumonia. In fact, researchers seem to infer that *anything* which badly compromises an immune system may elicit this disease.

This is why a correct assessment of pneumocystis in 1980 should have been, simply: Pneumocystis is moving into different populations; what immunosuppressive factors might be involved? Malnutrition, toxic drugs? Repeated episodes of sexual diseases? The hunt for one unique viral cause was really a bizarre departure from obvious precedent.

In the years 1976 to 1983, the Mayo Clinic recorded 53 cases of pneumocystis. The underlying conditions judged to be responsible were leukemia (15 patients), lymphoma (9 patients), malignancies (5 patients), AIDS (2 patients), inflammatory diseases treated with corticosterioids (16 patients).

In September, 1975, Walter Hughes, of St. Jude's Research Hospital, published a current-status paper on pneumocystis, in *Critical Reviews in Clinical Laboratory Sciences*. He assembled a much longer list of factors which could predispose a person to pneumocystis. The list included thymic displasia, hypoglycemia, cryptococcus, tuberculosis, and protein-calorie malnutrition.

Today a person led to developing pneumocystis pneumonia because of one of the above conditions Hughes lists would be called an AIDS patient. This would wrongly shift the blame for pneumocystis to the HIV virus.

Other researchers have pointed out that severe malnutrition can underlie pneumocystis. As mentioned earlier, some full-time junkies and alcoholics are known for their inability to pay for, or their chronic disinterest in food. Today were, say, an alcoholic to develop pneumocystis the diagnosis would be AIDS, HIV, and the whole ball of wax – not (correctly) pneumocystis stemming from alcohol and malnutrition.

Pneumocystis pneumonia has moved into new populations since 1977, but people have been dying of it, because of malnutrition[2], since World War Two. In fact, following the War, epidemics were seen in Europe, mainly in infants.

Hughes summarizes: "In Leipzig, 1000 cases were seen between 1945 and 1953. During the period from 1953 to 1957, 2000 cases were registered in Czechoslovakia, with 412 cases confirmed at autopsy . . . The first recognized case of P. carinii pneumonia (pneumocystis) in the United States was reported in 1956. *Since then, an increasing number of cases have occurred from year to year.*" (Emphasis added.)

Hughes then points out that there are no complete figures for pneumocystis in the U.S., but that, since 1967, the CDC has controlled the use of pentamidine, a specific pneumocystis drug. Therefore, by examining records of physicians' requests for the drug, an estimate of pneumocystis cases can be made.

"Over a three-year period from 1967 through 1970, 194 confirmed cases were recorded. However, in the year 1973 (5 years before the first diagnosed case of AIDS–author), the drug was dispensed to treat 527 proven or suspect cases of P. carinii pneumonitis. This may indicate an increase in prevalence rate because of the more extensive use of immunosuppressive (drug) therapy, prolonged survival of compromised hosts, or greater astuteness in the recognition of the infection."

There begins to be a very strange story here. First, it is clear that pneumocystis is not a new disease. Second, it was already increasing, from 1956 on. The question is, why did it begin to proliferate in new populations around 1977? According to Walter Hughes' analysis,

---

2 See RK Chandra *J. Pediatrics*, vol. 81, 1972, p. 1194 for background on undernutrition and immunocompetence. See also his letter to *Current Contents*, vol. 30, p. 15, June 1, 1987. Researchers turned up, in the early and mid-1970s, many cases of pneumocystis among undernourished children in Vietnam and Iran. It was generally understood at the time that pneumocystis was being overlooked internationally in the Third World, among children, and that it was mainly caused by malnutrition. See *JAMA*, March 1975, v. 231, p. 1190, "Mission to Saigon--An Alert for PCP (Pneumocystis)," Redman.

there could be a number of factors involved. Researchers concur that immunosuppressive drug therapy is a strong factor in causing the pneumocystis protozoa to come to the fore and instigate virulent disease. But does the medical profession have a monopoly on immunosuppressive drugs?

How far do you have to stretch to conclude that a wide spectrum of drugs used in concert in the gay community – antibiotics, speed, cocaine, ethyl chloride, heroin, poppers, MDA, quaaludes, valium, LSD, designer compounds – could rank as "immunosuppressive drug therapy?"

Not very far.

Remember, pneumocystis, by definition, is sufficient for a diagnosis of AIDS.

The rush to call hospitalized 1980 gay pneumocystis patients "previously healthy," and then to undertake a viral quest for the cause of their immune-suppression, leaving obvious background drug (and other) factors in the dust, has to rank as one of the most bizarre moves in the history of medicine.

There is other interesting commentary in the literature on pneumocystis. In 1971, Peter Rosen *et al* undertook a study of 20 New York pneumocystis patients.[3] Rosen concluded that "the clinical presentation of Pneumocystis infection may vary from fulminant to inapparent pneumonia and may be masked by preexistent pulmonary disease."

In other words, it can be hard to find. So it wouldn't be surprising if the disease, even in 1971, was being underreported. Rosen goes on to make the point that, indeed, as of 1971, there were no methods of testing blood for pneumocystis or isolating the microbe itself.

He also says, "Interest in the specific diagnosis of pneumocystis carinii pneumonia has been heightened in recent years by the therapeutic success with pentamidine isothionate."

It's not hard to piece together a simple story here. In the 1970s, the incidence of pneumocystis cases began rising partly because weakened cancer patients, many treated with increasingly toxic immuno-

---

[3] October, 1972, *The American Journal of Medicine*, vol. 53. p. 428.

suppressant drugs, were ripe for infection by ordinarily benign opportunistic organisms. Like pneumocystis. Doctors felt they had a drug to treat this pneumocystis pneumonia: pentamidine. The search continued for a better way to diagnose pneumocystis. Between 1977-80, it was found and took hold in hospitals: Percutaneous lung aspirate. From that point on, armed with a sensitive test, more cases began to be diagnosed. More pentamidine was used to treat them.

Many doctors are not aware of this story.

I spoke with a doctor who was familiar with increasing pneumocystis cases at Georgia's Eugene Talmadge Hospital in 1977, and also pneumocystis at St. Jude's hospital. "They were seeing five cases of pneumocystis a month in children at St. Jude's. They were all cancer patients, most with leukemia, some with solid tumors. The pneumocystis seemed to be arising both from the cancers and from the cancer drug-therapy. They were seeing some pneumocystis when the kids were first admitted, before any drug therapy was done," he said.

I asked this doctor if he would attribute the post-1977 increase in Talmadge pneumocystis to the introduction of diagnosis by percutaneous lung aspirate. "Yes," he said. He also told me that prior to this new 1977 method of diagnosing pneumocystis, the only method used at Talmadge was autopsy after death. Autopsy, of course, wasn't done on all patients who died from pneumocystis.

If autopsy was the primary method of diagnosing pneumocystis at Talmadge before 1977, then, afterward, with new diagnostic methods gradually being introduced – lung aspirate, broncheal lavage (which requires no hole made in the lung), and finally, today, fiberoptic bronchoscopy – the numbers of cases being located by these new, more sensitive techniques would naturally go up.

I then said, "It must be hard, if autopsy used to be a prominent method of diagnosis, to now say why pneumocystis cases *are* on the rise. We do have these new sensitive diagnostic tests, after all."

"It's a complex question," the doctor said. "There are variables. One is the frequency of autopsy that was being done (prior to 1977). Another is the new techniques of diagnosing pneumocystis that have gradually come along since 1977. The other is AIDS . . . With AIDS, we're much more aware of the possibility that there is pneumocystis (to find). So we're sensitive to testing for it."

What does it all add up to?

It seems apparent that the numbers of "pre-AIDS" pneumocystis cases have been underestimated, both because of less reliable diagnostic methods and because doctors were less alerted and disposed to look for them.

Although there is a long list of a) disease, b) malnutritive and c) chemical factors which can make the immunosuppressive bed in which pneumocystis will turn virulent, the CDC has severely ignored these factors, instead pushing HIV into the limelight as the "new" agent.

In particular, the extraordinary mix of medical and recreational drug-taking which, like immunosuppressive chemotherapy, could dispose toward pneumocystis, is written out of the AIDS equation.

People whose health is compromised, but still very reversible are not being told *how* significant these drug factors are in their lives. That is criminal.

A good example of AIDS-related research which has not floated to the top of the NIH research ladder is a paper by Peter Walzer et al, in the December 1984 *Infection and Immunity*. Walzer explores the possibility, in rats, that antibiotics can increase the disposition toward pneumocystis.

Walzer states, "Rats that were administered corticosteroids, a low-protein diet, and tetracycline spontaneously developed P. carinii pneumonia within ca. 8 weeks through a mechanism of reactivation of latent infection."[4]

In the U.S. gay community, malnutrition, abuse of tetracycline and corticosteroids are frequently found as partners.

In 1973, a major symposium on pneumocystis was undertaken at the National Cancer Institute. Authors Hughes, Sanyal, and Price remarked on a feature of some pneumocystis cases: ". . . patients with pneumocystis carinii pneumonia were underweight and had hy-

---

[4] See Author's Note, page v.

poproteinemia (protein calorie malnutrition) . . ." Malnutrition, a frequent partner of pneumocystis.

The bottom lines?

1. Pneumocystis can apparently occur from any severe form of immunosuppression: anemia, malnutrition, protein-calorie deficiency, toxic drugs, etc. The history of the disease was ignored, and still is, in rendering a diagnosis of "AIDS due to HIV."

2. If the Georgian doctor learned there were 60 cases of pneumocystis a year at St. Jude's hospital in the early and mid 1970s, how many cases were being seen (and missed) at hospitals all over the U.S.? There have been 32,000 cases of pneumocystis reported as AIDS since 1978. There is no CDC breakdown by year. The average would be about 3,000 cases a year. If 50 U.S. hospitals in the early 1970s had 60 cases a year, like St. Jude's, that would equal the current levels of "AIDS" pneumocystis.

(The CDC keeps *no* numbers on current "non-AIDS" pneumocystis cases).

3. Every person diagnosed with pneumocystis should be interviewed extensively by a good physician to determine the sources of immunosuppression *in his case.* Unfortunately, most physicians in this country are unable to assess the results of such an interview, since they have no knowledge of immunosuppressive drugs, medical or street-type, beyond a very parochial range. Furthermore, they frequently, under a variety of orthodox assurances, practice immunotoxic medicine. Blind spot.

4. To point out, in defense of an infectious viral theory of AIDS, that many gay men have developed pneumocystis since 1977, is only to establish the probability that, in gay communities, certain common immunosuppressive factors have been present. Drugs, STDs, for example.

Drugs like poppers and MDA and (vastly overused) antibiotics and corticosteroids immediately come to mind. Not a virus.

CHAPTER FOURTEEN

KAPOSI'S SARCOMA

Researchers have attempted to bolster the idea that AIDS is an infectious global epidemic, by linking Kaposi's sarcoma, one of its main symptoms, to both Africa and the U.S. But does the link hold?

Most researchers say Kaposi's sarcoma is a cancer of the blood vessels. It manifests on the skin or inside the body. Beginning as pink, red, or violet spots, or raised marks, it progresses to dark blue or purple-brown lesions, nodules or plaques.

Perhaps 30% of the time, it is found in the lungs, where it can be difficult to differentiate from pneumocystis pneumonia. When it affects the gastrointestinal tract, the major complication is bleeding.

At one time, about 30% of people diagnosed with AIDS in America had Kaposi. That percentage has steadily diminished in the last two years, according to CDC reports.

The public is not aware that there are at least three types of Kaposi. The so-called classical type is found in people of Eastern European and Mediterranean origins. It affects older people, is "indolent," as they say, has a protracted course, and the people who have it seem to live with it and die of natural causes.

Then there is endemic Kaposi, found in certain areas of Africa, particularly in Kenya, Tanzania, and Zaire. It has probably always existed in these regions. A person who has it usually suffers no ill effects, but after years it can suddenly flare up and become progressive.

Finally there is what is referred to as aggressive or epidemic Kaposi. This is the form found in the United States, which began to proliferate around 1980, particularly among gay men. It is generally agreed that some immune-depression accompanies this form. A number of researchers feel that the CMV virus is connected with aggressive Kaposi – perhaps through repeated infection by sex with a number of partners. And as mentioned earlier, inhalant nitrite drugs have also been proposed as a major cause.   One of the principal reasons black Africans and Europeans/Americans diagnosed with AIDS were connected was because Kaposi was found in all these groups. But which types of Kaposi?   That's not easy to answer once you scratch the surface.   Therefore, the whole Africa-U.S. Kaposi connection isn't solid.

In the June 1985 *Annals of Internal Medicine*, AA Otu describes the symptoms of traditional Kaposi in Nigeria: Large fungated tumors on the limbs, "massive lymphoedema," gangrene which ends up with amputation of the feet and legs. Otu also says that no patient with this type of Kaposi has been known to be an IV drug user, homosexual, or hemophiliac.

He concludes: "No increase in the prevalence of Kaposi has been seen over the last decade and no epidemiological data exist that show a change in the pattern of the disease during the same period. No patient with the acquired immune deficiency syndrome has been seen here."

Otu is saying there is a fourth manifestation of Kaposi which has existed traditionally in Nigeria, is virulent, and has nothing to do with AIDS. If so, this would throw cold water on the scenario which has it that aggressive Kaposi, as a new phenomenon, sprang up in Africa and the U.S. more or less simultaneously.

Bijan Safai, a well-know Kaposi researcher, points out that in the new epidemic form of Kaposi in the U.S., there is resemblance to a type of lymphadenopathy-associated Kaposi seen in African children. But is that African Kaposi new? Apparently not. This infection of children would possibly constitute a fifth type of Kaposi.

KR Oates, in *Family Practice*, June, 1986, states that in northeast Zaire, at the Centre Medical Evangelique Hospital in Nyankunde, which serves a population of 500,000, 15% of all malignancies are from Kaposi's sarcoma. This percentage has not changed in thirteen years – which would tend to mitigate against the idea of a new epidemic (AIDS-associated) Kaposi in that region.

The Uganda Cancer Institute, between October, 1983, and December, 1984, reported seeing only 4 Ugandans with Kaposi's sarcoma. I haven't been able to locate published studies which cover later periods, but I have been told by a Ugandan physician that Kaposi is rare in Uganda, to this day.

In general, AIDS information from Africa is very spotty, and people with one AIDS theory or another use reports which suit their fancy. For example, last May 11 (1987) the *London Times* ran a piece in which WHO health workers out of Geneva were predicting 75 million cases of full-blown AIDS in southern Africa, within five years. Place next to this the official statistics on African AIDS cases. As of October, 1987, the count was about 5000 AIDS cases on the whole continent.

Renee Sabatier, writing in the December, 1987, *Western Journal of Medicine,* points out that *Fodor's Guide to Kenya,* for vacationers, contains the cautionary statement, "Doctors speculate that in some African countries the (AIDS) infection rate may be 30% of the total population." Sabatier then adds, "There are no data to support such an assertion from any of the AIDS-affected African counties, least of all from Kenya . . ."

Based on HIV blood testing (inaccurate to say the least), this so-called "HIV infection" becomes a weapon of discouragement to tourists. Popular wisdom has it that African nations are dying, falling apart from AIDS, yet here, with Sabatier, we have contradictory information. You would think Africa was on Mars.

Back in America, there have been cases of Kaposi reported after immunosuppressive drug therapy. Kaposi has also been brought on by the steroid prednisone, and was reversed in one instance after discontinuing that drug. A case has also been reported in which a man developed KS after long-term use of sulfamide drugs.

In one USA study during which 24 postmortems of Kaposi patients were done, CMV virus was found to have been present in 75% of these people.

In other words, it is *quite* possible that the Kaposi sarcoma in the U.S. and African are different from one another – in the sense that they don't represent manifestations of one epidemic.

As I say, just trying to get a line on the incidence and types of Kaposi in Africa is difficult. Is what some clinicians there report as a new aggressive form the same as the U.S. version? Is it widespread?

Is it really an old, traditional form found in greater numbers now because of more surveillance owing to the publicity AIDS is getting?

A federal researcher recently said to me, "There are the lumpers and the splitters. The lumpers lump infections together (calling them AIDS), and the splitters break them down into separate diseases. In Africa, " he said, "we need more people who are willing to be splitters."

In America, NIH, CDC, the whole department of Health and Human Services, and in the world arena, the World Health Organization, are lumpers. They have welded together an image of a demonic, singular entity which is threatening all good folk, and they are stirring up the troops to do battle with HIV.

Once this battle has been enjoined, critics are of course ignored. There is no room for dissenters. The march to victory must proceed. The air of hysteria must be preserved.

Kaposi's sarcoma, the second most prevalent symptom of AIDS, may have an important, unexplored connection to the use of poppers in the U.S.; and efforts to tie together the disease in Africa and the U.S. fall far short of good science.

Those who try to use Kaposi as evidence for the global infectiousness of HIV-caused disease are relying on oversimplified imagery.

CHAPTER FIFTEEN

AN INTERVIEW WITH A MOLECULAR BIOLOGIST: DOES HIV CAUSE AIDS?

The following interview with a respected molecular biologist was done in the winter of 1988. As publication of this book neared, he decided *not* to go on the record with his remarks, and so I deleted his name from these pages. The alternative would have been to change certain parts of our conversation, and I refused to do that.

It is important to understand that at no time did this scientist retract anything he said. Nor did he feel, some months after our conversation, that the considerable force of his remarks needed tempering because of recent research developments concerning AIDS. On the contrary, he has become more convinced than ever that HIV has not been proven to cause human disease.

He had his own personal reasons for removing his name from this interview. They concerned how he would be judged by his peers, most of whom are utterly convinced that HIV is the central disease-agent of our time–though, he told me, "I can't figure out for the life of me why they think so. Has the quality of research deteriorated so badly? Let me answer my own question. Yes."

In this, and the next conversation with Peter Duesberg, both men maintain: Not only is HIV unproven as the cause of AIDS, it is latent, dormant, it lies around without replicating, without spreading. There is no evidence, either, that it destroys human cells in the body. There is no conclusive evidence that it gives rise to indirect mechanisms which in turn destroy cells or harm the body. When the actual virus can be found in a person who has been diagnosed with AIDS, its concentration (titer) is so low that special lab procedures have to be used to induce it to grow in a dish, outside the body, so that *then* it can be detected at all. It exists in so few cells that even if it did destroy them, the result would be "like a pinprick."

It is important to note that, whether one agrees or disagrees with the way these two scientists characterize the personality of HIV, that virus is still unproven as the cause of disease.

Q: You've read a great many professional papers written on the subject of AIDS. What is their general quality?

A: Their general quality is poor. Poor, relative to good virology. Poor, relative to papers with well assembled statistics. Poor compared with rational thought.

Q: Any speculation as to why that is?

A: It's a very important epidemic.

Q: I don't understand.

A: It's an easy field in which to get money to do experiments. It's an easy field to publish in. People tend to publish hastily.

Q: Why are so many researchers convinced that HIV causes AIDS?

A: You mean people who work on HIV? I don't know why they think it causes AIDS. I think there's a lot of circumstantial evidence you can use to convince yourself that what you're working on is important, is worth doing. There's a tremendous amount of authoritarianism in science. When everyone is telling you that this is so (HIV causes AIDS), it's easy to convince yourself that, indeed, it must be so, otherwise how could all these people be working on it?

You're a retrovirologist. You're told by everybody that there is transfusion-AIDS and that it's now been stopped. That there is pediatric AIDS. That there are cohort studies in which it's known that AIDS is transmissible. You've been told that by the head of the CDC, by the head of the Allergy and Infectious Diseases unit and you're getting more grant money than you've had in ten years, to work on this virus. And every time you find something, it's immediately publishable, in the best journals. So why should you not believe it? Why should you pay attention to a man like Peter Duesberg who comes along and says, 'Wait a minute, hold on here, let's relook at all this data that you believe in.' In fact, when you look at what you believe about AIDS, you find that it's all quite fatuous. There is no hard evidence (that HIV causes AIDS). But few people are going to reverse their field.

Q: We hear that once upon a time, people used to debate issues like HIV seriously, freely, in journals. They didn't ignore these issues.

A: There has never been a time before this when medical research and basic biological research were both connected to the money machine. The fundamental change is that now biology is a for-profit science. Yearly, the directory of biotechnology companies grows.

Q: Was there really a period when issues of biology were debated freely and openly?

A: Yes. I grew up in molecular biology at a time when theories were constantly debated in the journals. This is what molecular biology was. The debate about whether there in fact existed a repressor molecule, debates about specific initiation factors, how E-coli DNA replication proceeded, whether it proceeded from one origin or several origins. People of considerable talent debated these issues, with good experimental data. Whether transforming viruses had particular oncogenes or not. Pretty good debate. Still going on in one form or another.

The argument that you hear from the AIDS establishment – "Oh my God, what would have happened if AIDS occurred twenty years ago when we didn't have the techniques we have today, it would have wiped out the universe" – I turn that around. In some ways I would rather have seen AIDS twenty years ago. When it would have been dealt with by more orthodox medical practices and it would be over with.

Q: People say they've proved AIDS is transmissible.

A: If one tries to differentiate transmissibility of the disease from transmissibility of the virus, it's extraordinarily easy to do. Once you remove the equation that transmission of the virus equals transmission of the disease, AIDS does not look like a terribly transmissible disease anymore.

Q: In other words, if you don't make the assumption that HIV causes AIDS, all you have is the transmission of this interesting but possibly harmless virus.

A: That's right. The disease itself does not appear terribly transmissible . . . the transmissibility within a cohort, when studied, is always within cohorts that are engaging in precisely the same kind of activity, so it's impossible to say that X gave it to Y who gave it to Z. All you know is that X, Y, and Z were doing the same thing, and X, Y, and Z came down with the same peculiar set of infections.

Q: And one thing they were doing was having sex with each other in, say, the case of the gay community.

A: That's one of the things they were doing. They were doing a whole bunch of other things . . . under the umbrella of ingesting large numbers of potent chemicals.

And in the other (risk) groups, who knows what the AIDS is? One looks at transfusion AIDS, and in the time between 1978 and 1983, there were millions of transfusions in the U.S., when the blood supply was not being screened, was not being scrutinized, and should have contained the largest amount of this virus at any time in "the epidemic's history." And out of those millions of transfusions, there were 400 cases of transfusion-related AIDS. And of that 400, only a small fraction of them are really described in the medical literature, as to their symptoms, and in none of them does one know the HIV (status) of the recipient *before* the transfusion. Again, these are whole-blood transfusions. They could have gotten some nasty combination of things (other than HIV) from the blood which gave them their AIDS. If you want to be hard core about it, tranfusing whole blood doesn't exclude *anything* else (as a possible cause of subsequent disease).

Q: I have the picture that only a few people control the necessary equipment to do research on HIV.

A: No. Nothing special about that at all.[1]

Q: This equipment is available to lots of people.

A: Oh yes. Lots and lots of people are working on HIV. Whole companies have been founded on it.

---

[1] Some sources state that Robert Gallo has long controlled who gets the HIV virus for study and research purposes.

Q: A few, but not all studies, show that HIV antibodies are found more often in people with AIDS, or people in so called high risk groups, than in people from low risk groups. Why?

A: Because the virus is hard to transmit. Hard to cause even a sign that it has been present in the body. It would be more likely to show up in people whose immune systems were shot. Probably, on the whole, there are more people in high risk groups whose immune systems are already compromised.

Q: What would have to be shown to say that HIV causes AIDS?

A: What would be convincing to me? A chimpanzee succumbing to AIDS. That would make me go back and look at the other arguments and say, well, there's something going on we just don't understand. Also (to convince me) a demonstration that the virus has an active site of replication[2] (in the human body), at some concealed site that we don't really know about. And that its replication in that spot is somehow destructive to T-helper cells. Also (to convince me), the demonstration of a plausible mechanism to explain latency of the virus.[3]

Q: You mean plausible genetic mechanisms?

A: Genetic, physiological, biochemical, immunological – I don't care. Something. Anything. Anything that made the slightest bit of biological sense. I don't see it. And I think the (HIV) virus is really well known. There isn't a single secret in the genome (genetic structure). No new gene waiting there to come out. There's hard evidence that says HIV only behaves in a particular way. Like every other retrovirus, extremely latent, extremely inactive . . . not killing the human cell in which it's expressing (its) genes.

HIV is in people with symptoms, and in people without symptoms. If there is a secret site where it really is replicating, it seems to

---

[2] Several researchers are coming to the conclusion that HIV does not actively and aggressively replicate, does not produce more and more of itself in the body.
[3] Latency refers to the initial period of months, or years, during which HIV supposedly lives in the body without causing measurable harm, after which it is said to become active and virulent.

me one should have been able to detect that by now, with the kind of scrutiny that has gone on.

Q: How could a fantasy arise that HIV was replicating to begin with?

A: It was just taken as an assumption, all the way along, and when the data began to show that it wasn't so, that data was just ignored. People said, "Well, we know it's causing the disease, and when we understand more about its behavior, we'll understand this replicating business too. This too shall come to pass." It's a myth that's constantly being provided the world through Gallo and Fauci and others who claim that this is the most complicated retrovirus in the history of the universe. "With more study we'll understand everything, it's so peculiar, how it behaves, how it causes this disease, but don't worry, we'll figure it out."

But all the things that are peculiar about it are things that would make you look at it and say, Gee, this virus is not a pathogen! It doesn't do anything. Humans make a perfectly good antibody response to it; in fact it's so good, maybe that's why the virus is so latent (harmless).

Q: Recently, Gallo said animal models[4] for smallpox and tuberculosis never existed either, and used that as a reason for ignoring the fact that chimps don't get AIDS.

A: I'm not sure about tuberculosis. Smallpox will not infect chimpanzees. But there is a very virulent monkeypox which is an exact animal model for human smallpox.

Simian viruses, though, are lousy models for human AIDS. They're said to be good models, but nobody really believes they're good models, because of the following reasons: It is not a disease (monkey AIDS) that occurs in the wild. It only occurs in caged monkeys. It can only be given to these monkeys by injecting them with high doses of the virus at a time when their immune systems are rather poorly developed, immature. The onset of the immunodeficiency is rapid, there is an accompanying viremia, the opportunistic

---

[4] Refers to the step in fulfilling Koch's postulates, in which animals are injected with a germ thought to cause a disease, to see if all the symptoms develop in them.

infections are quick, and very lethal. The whole thing is over quickly. Take those things and say, how much of that looks like AIDS? Plus the (simian) virus itself is very unrelated to HIV. How much of a model is that for human AIDS? It's a terrible model, in all of its aspects.[5]

Q: What about the people who argue that, say, viruses like sheep visna are good comparisons for HIV? Visna is supposed to be a latent virus that lies around for a long time in sheep and then causes brain rot that kills them.

A: That's another one of those viruses . . . when you have the disease, you can't find the virus anymore.

Q: You mean it's like HIV in that respect.

A: Yes. Arguing about visna on behalf of AIDS is assuming that the data about visna is understood. That we understand how this (sheep disease) happens. That we understand how a sheep can get infected and 20 years later, ten years later, can develop this neuro-encephalopathy. The whole field of slow viruses cannot be held up (as an example for AIDS). Some of those viruses don't even exist. They only exist in the journals. Like kuru virus. It's highly specious.

Q: In other words, you're saying, since we don't understand how visna plays a role in malignant sheep disease, then there's no way to make a parallel to HIV.

A: Yes. Visna is a case in which there isn't (virus production). When the animal dies, you can't find the virus anymore.

To explain HIV latency by visna latency is imagining you understand visna latency.

Q: Do you think there are researchers out there, people who are thinking, "I'd really like to say in public I agree with Duesberg, but I don't want to. I shouldn't."

A: There must be. Duesberg will make it that much more difficult for figures to be fudged in the future, to perhaps keep an epidemic going that really doesn't exist, and to continue to use the fear

---

5 Also, in order to get microbes to infect monkeys, the animals may be radiated or dosed with chemical toxins, both of which weaken their immune systems. Such procedures would further disqualify animal-model analogies to human AIDS.

that any moment now we're all going to get it (AIDS); to manipulate people, which I think is the overriding political interest, in AIDS. If Duesberg is right . . . then the imagined numbers of cases will not develop. Evidently, they've not developed in Haiti. I can't find anybody who has any real information on what's happened to the 200,000 cases that were supposed to develop in Haiti by now.

The AIDS literature is full of screw-ups. Papers that are published with great authority that are baloney. You look at the data and it's unbelievable, the conclusions that are drawn from them: Papers about homologies between AIDS protein and other proteins. The gene experiments with HIV, which tell you nothing about the way these HIV genes function in the body, in the human organism. You're talking about a virus (HIV) that doesn't *do* anything, except in Gallo's H9-line (a laboratory cell-line used to culture HIV and make it grow). He probably proclaims HIV grows in this cell-line of his better than in any cell-line in the world, that that's why he can study it better than anyone else can. Blithely overlooking the fact that he's got a cell-line infected by HIV, making more HIV, making more of this "deadly" virus than any cell-line known to man. And yet this "deadly" virus doesn't kill these cells it's growing in. Bizarre.

It became very fashionable at some point to say that if you had a disease and from the patient you simply isolated a retrovirus (a class of virus to which HIV belongs), the retrovirus was automatically the cause of the disease. That set the stage for isolating a retrovirus from AIDS patients and calling it the cause of the disease.

Q: Fashionable?

A: Yes.

This interview suggests one of the reasons researchers don't want to debate anti-HIV people in any serious way, which is to say in professional journals. Their critique of HIV has roots in deeper criticisms of virology that have to do with unwarranted assumptions about the latency of certain animal viruses. That would move the debate back over twenty to thirty years of significant biological research and throw doubt on the value of it.

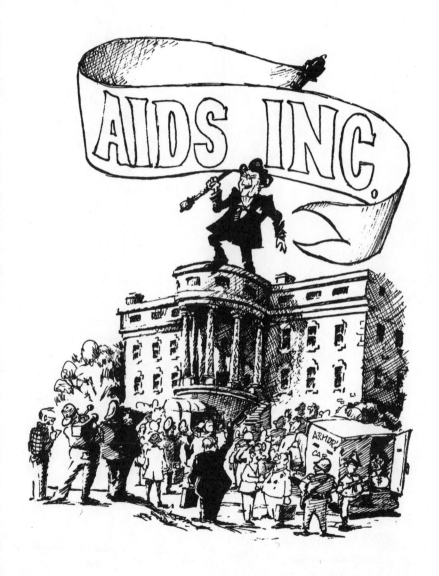

CHAPTER SIXTEEN

AN INTERVIEW WITH PETER DUESBERG:
DOES HIV CAUSE AIDS?

Peter Duesberg, a molecular biologist at the University of California at Berkeley, was recently on sabbatical at the National Institutes of Health in Maryland.[1] There he resided among the leading AIDS researchers of the day. Duesberg was also a key researcher during the war on cancer, when he worked side by side with people who are now top AIDS investigators. Including Robert Gallo, an old friend of his. Gallo is the co-discoverer of HIV.

Duesberg asserts that HIV is not the cause of AIDS.

To understand the import of that conviction, one has to understand that the National Institutes of Health (NIH) have taken in several hundred million dollars in a quest to cure AIDS. That money, the commitment to a cure, all hang on the one breakthrough the medical research establishment claims: The discovery of the AIDS virus, HIV.

On March 1, 1987, *Cancer Research,* a venerable professional journal, published Peter Duesberg's paper on the subject of HIV. Since then, some sense of challenge has entered the scene. Things are not quite what they were. Several researchers, incognito, have approached Duesberg and privately told him they agree with his assessment that the medical-research establishment has failed to prove HIV is the AIDS virus – that in fact, Duesberg was pointing out the obvious: the emperor had no clothes.

What follows is an interview excerpted and edited from several conversations with Professor Duesberg, during the summer of 1987 and the winter of 1988.

Q: From what I gather, you are saying that HIV is really an inactive virus, not aggressive at all.

---

[1] During the summer of 1987.

A: That's right. It infects a very, very small percentage of cells, in low concentrations. One in 10,000, one in 100,000 cells. The whole class to which it belongs – retroviruses – are really very poor candidates for a disease like AIDS.

Q: Certainly if what you say is true, Robert Gallo and others know it too. I mean, if it's ordinary information that any biologist would know . . .

A: You have to be at NIH to see how they think. They're very, very concerned with the next research step. The step that comes after what they've just discovered. You could remind them that the kind of virus they're studying, HIV, just doesn't really qualify to cause a disease like AIDS, and they would understand what you were saying, and they might even agree with you, as far as general principles were concerned. But then they'd turn around and go right back to working on what they were doing before they talked to you.

Q: Do you see Robert Gallo at NIH?

A: I've known him for a long time. He doesn't want to talk about my paper (in *Cancer Research*). He says, "With friends like you, who needs enemies."

Q: Do people ask him about your paper?

A: People do, yes. It annoys him. He doesn't want to get into a debate about it, about HIV. I did give a seminar recently. Sabin (the inventor of the oral polio vaccine) got up there and praised my paper. That was nice. He said it deserved attention.

Q: Why is Robert Gallo on top of the heap, leading the war on AIDS?

A: I really don't know.

Q: In your paper, *Retroviruses as Carcinogens and Pathogens: Expectation and Reality*, you say, 'It is concluded that AIDS virus is not sufficient to cause AIDS and that there is no evidence, besides its presence in a latent form, that it is necessary for AIDS.' In other words, although the HIV virus is present in a proportion of AIDS patients, Gallo and others have not proved that it causes the disease.

A: Many AIDS patients have the herpes virus too, but no one is saying herpes causes AIDS.

Q: We see, on television, what are possibly computerized models of HIV attacking human cells and forcing them to reproduce copies of itself and in general doing a great deal of damage. Are these simulations?

A: Yes. HIV will enter a host cell, but the devastation part – I'm not saying the television depiction is intentionally phony, but it's not a true picture.

Q: Do we definitely know that AIDS is a viral disease?

A: No.

Q: Could HIV possibly be affecting the thymus, where the immune-system's T-cells are generated? Could HIV be destroying the immune system that way?

A: It's theoretically possible, I suppose, but no evidence exists that that's happening. If HIV attacked the thymus, you'd see a reservoir of it, a large concentration of it at some point in the thymus. We haven't seen that.

Q: If you were running AIDS research, what major change would you make – aside from rolling back the assumption that HIV is the cause? It seems to me that your paper makes some very sweeping criticisms of the way that laboratory research, in general, is carried on. Artificial high titers being introduced, for example, to make virulent effects where none would exist in real life, in the human body.

A: I would take AIDS research from the lab much more into the clinical situation. See what patients are showing. What are their signs. I would look at patients much more. Our instrumentation these days is so sensitive. So we have a tendency to remove ourselves from real life.

Q: At the top of the AIDS research establishment, there is a great deal of politics, at least in the sense that you have to claim you have a major discovery like HIV and a cure on the way, in order to justify millions of research dollars. That could warp your scientific attitude.

A: It's very hard to talk to a person who has a contract with a drug company in his pocket. How do you know that he's telling you the truth? Times have changed. This is high-stakes science, financially.

Q: Would it be correct to say that HIV is *associated* with AIDS?

A: What is associated with AIDS is *antibodies* to HIV. Antibodies are a sign that you've successfully dealt with a virus, not a prognosis of disease. A titer (detectable concentration) of HIV has *never been reported* yet in one patient, in a paper on AIDS. Gallo, Levy, and Montagnier say they can't isolate HIV itself in more than 50% of the cases.

We have made up our minds much too early. We should go back and define what we mean by the disease. We talk about it as if it is *the* disease, a disease entity. It is a combination of symptoms which are highly heterogeneous and have little to do with each other.

Q: In Africa, they say HIV infects women and men on an equal basis.

A: So far as Africa is concerned, we don't even know what is going on in the U.S. Africa doesn't help make things clear. Gallo and a few others go over there with their HIV antibody test kits, they bring home a few pictures of people dying, and they say the whole continent is going under. Meanwhile, about 4000 cases of AIDS have been reported in Africa.

Q: You're saying that retroviruses like HIV are easy to find with the hi-tech equipment at the disposal of virologists today. That, therefore, their mere discovery implies nothing about whether these viruses cause disease.

A: There is no mouse in this world that doesn't have at least 50 retroviruses in him as latent as the HIV virus. No chicken, no cow, no cat. We can now see, in the lab, a (viral) part in a billion (of cell-volume), or a part in ten billion. We are approaching physics. So I would amend Koch's postulates to say we have to see some biochemical activity out of a virus, in order to *start* imagining it might cause disease.

Koch and Pasteur, when they considered under what conditions a germ could cause disease, couldn't, of course, know anything about our present level of magnification. They would never have been able to see HIV. Koch was looking at somebody who was *loaded* with tuberculosis. Pasteur was looking at somebody who was *loaded* with rabies virus. What researchers today can do is great detective work (finding retroviruses), but it's clinically absurd. But that's all they can do. That's their skill. So they have to believe they're finding the cause of disease.

Q: So you're saying, in amendment to Koch's postulates, that a virus must be biochemically active.

A: Yes. It must be infecting more cells than the host can spare. Every month, half of your T-cells are new. So the HIV virus would have to infect a couple percent of them every day. It doesn't. You don't become demented from losing .1% of your brain cells. You don't become an AIDS patient from losing .01% of your T-cells . . . That's like a pin prick. HIV infects one out of 10,000, one out of 100,000 cells.

Q: One researcher has said he admits the HIV virus has a very unconventional pathology, but that's no reason to ignore the virus.

A: If we knew HIV caused disease, yes. But that question, in the case of AIDS, has never been proved.

Q: Certain researchers have used, as an anology to HIV, other animal viruses. For example, bovine leukemia virus, calling it the cause of bovine leukemia and stating that BLV can be isolated from both leukemic and normal cells.

A: But not one reference proved the BLV causes the leukemia, *only that the virus could be isolated*. There is an analogy to AIDS here. It is that BLV is consistently latent, even during leukemia, and there are large quantities of BLV-antibody. This argues precisely *against* a viral etiology of leukemia. Consistently latent (dormant) virus, good antibody responses – these factors describe what is commonly called immunization or vaccination. A healthy response.

If you inject newborns (animals) with BLV, you may get a wasting illness, but that is because these newborns are immune-tolerant (have unformed immune responses).

Q: In the July 6 *New York Native*, you said the following about the drug, AZT: "(To go ahead with AZT treatment under these circumstances) . . . to put it as kindly as possible, I think it's highly irresponsible . . . (AZT) is hell for the bone marrow . . . It kills normal cells quite, quite extensively   . . . AZT is a poison. It is cytotoxic. I think that giving it to people with AIDS is highly irresponsible . . . the drug is only going to hurt you."

A: That's right. And now they are giving it to people with no symptoms. It's supposed to prevent HIV from replicating, yet they can find no evidence that HIV is replicating in the first place.

Q: What would convince you that HIV played a role in AIDS?

A: If you could show it had some form of activity, some biochemical activity.

Q: If they can show that HIV infects just a few immune cells which then go crazy after 50 generations of carrying HIV as a latent virus – HIV suddenly erupts in these few cells and the cells then screw up the rest of the immune system . . . ?

A: This is like opening up some cyanide capsule. Goering had that in his tooth. You crack the capsule when things get too difficult and you're gone. If the virus could do that . . . but just *show* me the virus is biochemically active.

There's another theory that HIV isn't active, it just sends out one molecule to some kind of relay that explodes. You know, it's a signal that goes to a nuclear device in the thymus gland that explodes. I would really like to see that signal.

And if HIV is biochemically active, if they show me it makes protein RNA and DNA, then I would say it's time to consider it seriously – because that's what all other parasites have to do to get something done.

Second, I would like to see T-cells, or whatever it is – maybe they're moving to macrophages (as the seat of purported HIV infection) – I would have to see cells being killed (by HIV), not just .01% of them over five years. If you want to conquer a country, you can't do it by killing 5000 people every day when there are 100,000 new babies born every day.

Then the host (of HIV) would also have to be permissive. When you have antibodies (generated to HIV), the virus isn't going to succeed. The best time for all viruses to work is right away when you're a virgin. Before you generate that immune-response. But HIV doesn't do that.

If a chimp came down with so-called AIDS symptoms after being injected with HIV, I'd want to see what the virus was doing.

Q: If those symptoms took three years to develop in the chimp?

A: Anything with a long latent period is suspicious. Particularly if the long latent period follows the gaining of immunity. Of course, in lab experiments with animals, especially now with the hysteria about AIDS, researchers will forget to write down the titers of the virus they injected in the animals, or the fact that the animals are newborn and have no solid immune-response. In these cases, retroviruses can produce illnesses, yes, if you are using newborns and high titers of a virus. Then you get acute infection, which happens more quickly.

Of course, now they have about fifteen symptoms that are admissible as AIDS. Anything short of pregnancy, and I don't know, breast cancer, maybe. I mean, tell me what's not AIDS! Antibody positive, and you forget the keys to your car. I'm not making it up. In Florida, there was this young Cuban boy. He forgot the keys to his car several times. He couldn't remember where they were, and came to the hospital with some other problems. The doctor said, what are you doing? He said he was walking the streets. The doctor said, let's check you. He found the boy was antibody-positive to HIV and diagnosed him as having AIDS dementia. This case goes to the CDC as an AIDS statistic. What *is* AIDS? I think that's where we should start.

Q: You worked during the war on cancer in the special viral cancer project. Did you go from being converted to being disillusioned with the process of trying to prove cancer was transmitted by viruses?

A: Disillusioned is probably too strong a word. I went from being naive to being more realistic about it. It is not as important (viruses as agents of cancer) as I thought it was, as many people still think it is. I'm not as important as I thought I was. Or my work isn't. That includes a whole number of leading scientists right now: the Baltimores, the Weinbergs, the Varmuses, and the Gallos. Temin, even. Essex. Their reputations are based essentially on this view that retroviruses are significant candidates for carcinogens. That hasn't panned out. But it explains why there is generally so little criticism of the view that HIV (a retrovirus) causes AIDS. The view pleases all the old veterans of the virus-cancer program. They're all marching again. They used to be, essentially, on reserve. And now, all of a sudden, here's a windmill for them again. And they're attacking. So they get their boots, their uniforms, their tanks, and they're all ready to work on retroviruses. That's what they can do. These guys that used to be latent, somewhere in reserve, now they're marching. The old tune: retroviruses.

Retroviruses are all very similar. I mean, there are differences, but as far as pathology is concerned, you don't see a marker in one which is going to explain why it supposedly wakes up from sleep and becomes active. You may see markers in the gene structure that explain why one virus is a blonde and one is a brunette. But these are not clinically significant factors.

Q: Could AIDS vaccine research be dangerous in its potential effect on people?

A: I think the vaccine research is more silly than dangerous. Maybe the people doing the research could be dangerous, I don't know. On the one hand they say, look how wonderful we are, we're going to give you protection against HIV by producing antibodies in you. On the other hand, when people develop antibodies to HIV on their own and that is detected in a blood test, other people burn down their houses and people commit suicide.

Q: Robert Gallo says people have odd immune responses to the HIV virus which in turn destroy their own T-cells.

A: It's a hypothesis. He thinks antibodies to the virus would destroy the T-cells. I don't see the basis for the hypothesis. It doesn't seem to happen to the one to two million Americans who have antibodies to HIV. If people get AIDS, it doesn't happen either. I don't know of anything to support this hypothesis. It's one of the many great ideas of Dr. Gallo.

Q: Gallo says that even though HIV is present in low titers, it works to cause illness through indirect mechanisms like autoimmunity (the immune system attacking the body), or through

130

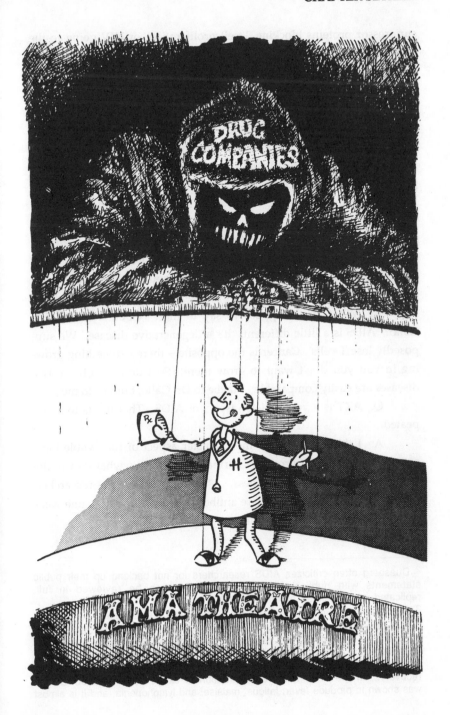

suppressor proteins blocking T-cell proliferation, or HIV going to the brain.

A: Again, another great idea for Dr. Gallo. I haven't seen a paper from him on autoimmunity. I don't know why autoimmunity should only affect risk groups like male homosexuals or IV drug users and not heterosexuals or girls. The suppressor proteins – another idea. If Dr. Gallo knows what they are, he should publish something about it.[2] Unfortunately, there's not much evidence for HIV going to the brain either. People have looked in brain cells and haven't found it. They've found it in blood cells in the brain, but very, very little.

Q: Gallo states, "Peter Duesberg doesn't understand latency. Do you think you get cancer in two weeks in nature . . . . With HTLV-1, the 1978 leukemia virus we discovered, you don't get cancer for twenty years."[3]

A: What am I suppose to say to that? Good morning, Dr. Gallo? AIDS is a little different. It's a degenerative disease. We supposedly lose T-cells. Cancer is the opposite – there's something growing in you you don't want to grow there. So I don't think the two diseases are easily comparable. Maybe to Dr. Gallo, but not to me.

Q: AZT is a very sinister aspect of AIDS. That needs to be repeated.

A: I think AZT is the most sinister aspect of this whole business. They're killing growing (normal) cells. That's what they're doing. That's very serious business. . . Hazeltine (Harvard researcher) proposed to treat babies that are antibody-positive (to HIV), one week with AZT, the other week with interferon[4] .

---

[2] Duesberg often criticizes AIDS researchers for not backing up their public statements with published papers which can then be reviewed in full, replicated, or challenged by other scientists.

[3] Gallo interview, *Spin* magazine, Feb. 1988, Anthony Liversidge.

[4] See Jan Vilcek, *Progress in Medical Virology*, vol. 30, 1984, p. 62: "Interferon is produced in the course of most common virus infections in man. It is likely that in many instances interferon production during an acute viral infection is beneficial as it may limit the spread of virus and promote recovery...On the other hand, administration of exogenous interferon to man was shown to produce fever, fatigue, malaise, and lymphopenia, and it is almost

Q: On February 20, 1988, you testified before the Presidential Commission on AIDS. A member of the Commission, Frank Lilly, criticized several points you made. For example, he said that HIV affects both heterosexuals and homosexuals, both men and women, when you look at the global picture. Therefore, it is not behaving any differently from any other virus.

A: Look, first of all, if there are reliable statistics to be found, they are in the U.S., not in other places. In the U.S., the CDC says that 92% of the AIDS patients in the U.S. are men. 92%. The remaining 8% are women and children. And then I want to know, instead of just saying these women have AIDS, what is the name of what they really had? Was it diarrhea, or dementia, or breast cancer, or did they forget briefly the name of their brother-in-law's cousin, or what? And then I want to know how many of these "AIDS" problems existed in a sample of women ten years before there was any such word, AIDS. And then I would subtract whatever *that* figure is from the 8% now, and we may have, for instance, three women that we are talking about now who supposedly have AIDS.

What I am talking about here, the extreme preference for men over women, is not the epidemiology of any infectious agent I know of. Microbes are not that picky.

Q: In Gallo's interview in *Spin* magazine, he kept saying, Duesberg is a funny guy. You have to know him. He's different. What is he talking about?

A: I think he means, I say what's on my mind. I don't mind the consequences. You have to understand what these researchers at NIH are like, the ones who believe in HIV. They have grown up with these viruses. It's the first thing they knew. That is usually very powerful in shaping your later attitudes, what you learn first. With these people, it was retroviruses. *They were taught from the beginning that they cause disease.* So it's an article of faith and it always

---

certain that similar symptoms seen in many common acute virus infections are, at least in part, due to the production of endogenous interferon."

The idea that interferon is unequivocally helpful is offset by strong dissent. In fact, the negative symptoms Vilcek mentions, which can occur from administering interferon, are Pre-AIDS symptoms. Yet there continue to be studies in which interferon is given to AIDS patients.

will be. NIH is like a military place, you know. In its attitude. They look at me, I'm from Berkeley, so they think I'm different. Free speech, all that. I work at a university, I speak my mind. At NIH, if you start asking questions in public about these viruses, you're out of a job. Retrovirology is also like religion. There are what, 700 million Catholics in the world? They all believe that Jesus was the son of God, but the proof is only circumstantial. It's the same thing at NIH with HIV.

Q: When they are alone, these researchers, do you think they express their doubts?

A: Sure. They have questions. They just don't want the public to know about these doubts.

CHAPTER SEVENTEEN

AIDS DEMENTIA AND THE PSYCHIATRISTS

I spoke with my anonymous doctor-friend in New York. The subject turned to AIDS dementia. Early symptoms, listed in journals, encompassed such behavior as being unable to keep track of the plot of a thick novel, forgetting appointment times, leg weakness.

Later on, these symptoms would supposedly develop into full-blown incoherence and mental confusion.

The dementia business was quite strange, to say the least, especially since some professionals in the field were maintaining that it may be the first or *only* manifestation of AIDS in some people.[1]

The doctor referred me to a journal article (*Science*, Feb. 5, 1988, vol. 239, p. 586). "Ask around," he said. "Ask a few people about that weird diagram in the article. It's supposed to be showing levels of HIV infection in the brain. I mean, this is the whole reason they're so confident these symptoms are really a form of AIDS. They say the dementia is caused by HIV attacking the brain."

I talked with a respected molecular biologist, and asked him what he thought about AIDS dementia and its recent depiction.

"Oh yes," he said. "That." He had seen it. "The diagram is supposed to depict the ups and downs, the different levels of HIV brain-infection during the course of dementia. *But no time-period is indicated, no numerical levels are shown. There are no numbers given at all*. It's absurd. The whole idea of connecting greater levels of HIV infection with progressively worse dementia falls completely short. The fact is, no one has found heavy concentrations of HIV in *any* AIDS patient. The concentrations are minute. Very, very minute."

---

[1] See *Arch. Neurol.* January, 1987, vol. 44, p. 65, RW Price et al.

My New York doctor had a good deal more to say about AIDS dementia. "Take one of the listed symptoms. Ataxia. It simply means failure or irregularity of muscle coordination. But you'll find in a medical dictionary there are a number of forms of ataxia. Alcoholic ataxia, Briquet's ataxia, Broca's ataxia. In fact, alcoholism can bring on most if not all the symptoms listed as AIDS dementia."

"You're saying this is a definitional shuffle?" I said. "A shell-game?"

"They're saying HIV virus in the brain causes these symptoms. But have they proved that? No. It's not even close."

"So all that's left is the symptoms."

"A whole bunch of them. They could be attributed to any number of causes. As a matter of fact, one cause is severe diarrhea. If you have diarrhea long enough, you get dehydrated. Then you lose electrolytes. And *that* can cause all sorts of mental symptoms. Confusion, disorientation, weird thoughts."

We then talked about the enlarged role of psychiatrists in AIDS, partly because of AIDS dementia.

"Every professional wants a piece of the pie," he said. "The psychiatrists are no exception. The easiest way to establish a role is to show that some AIDS symptoms belong in your bailiwick. Dementia is now listed as an AIDS indicator disease in the official definition. That means if you're diagnosed with it, you 'have' full-blown AIDS."

The doctor said there were other interesting aspects of the entrance of psychiatrists into AIDS.

In the counseling of patients, given the widespread opinion that AIDS is a terminal disease, the issues of suicide and euthanasia arise. Not just for those with advanced immune-suppression, but for those who have simply tested positive for exposure to the HIV virus. As the AIDS industry gathers steam – and I have several reports on this – patients are now being "permitted" to believe that the blood test is the only thing one needs to see in order to know whether death is inevitable.

There is now, in California, a measure on the ballot to allow euthanasia in terminal illness. Indications are that the insurance industry may eventually support such legislation. After all, the medical system is already feeling the considerable financial crunch of paying for hospitalization of AIDS patients.

"Dementia," the doctor said, "is an entry point into deciding that the AIDS patient is not competent to determine his future. Psychiatrists would be called in to make the diagnosis. They would also, at times, counsel AIDS patients who were suicidal. They would end up playing a role if euthanasia is made legal. The mix of declaring a patient mentally incompetent and discussing, at the same time, suicide/euthanasia could become volatile. As in, unduly influencing patients. Of course, some of those diagnosed with early AIDS dementia do go on to develop serious instability. They become incontinent, bed-ridden, unable to manage themselves. Some die. But all this is true with *any serious degenerative disease.*"

Yet one more opportunity, based on a list of mental symptoms, to use an unproven and emotionally devastating label, AIDS. To blame everything on HIV. To inflate AIDS case-statistics. To even suggest that suicide might not be a bad idea.

"Heavy drug use, exposure to combinations of chemicals could certainly produce what they call early signs of dementia," I said.

"Of course," the doctor said. "So could simply being diagnosed HIV positive."

I later obtained a copy of a booklet, *AIDS' Effect on the Brain*, published by the San Francisco-based AIDS Health Project, under the auspices of the University of California Regents. It contains an interesting section: "Some people with AIDS may become confused or show personality changes. These changes may be due to *direct* brain infection with the human immunodeficiency virus (HIV), the cause of AIDS. Or they may result from such causes as: anxiety, depression, medication, or a treatable illness related to AIDS.

"About half of those with AIDS or ARC develop signs of brain involvement during their illness. Many of these signs are due to a cause other than HIV infection in the brain. *Only a physician can diagnose the underlying cause of these changes. If a person with AIDS develops the problems described in this pamphlet, it is essential to seek medical evaluation.*" (Emphasis added.)

AIDS INC.

The idea that only a physician is competent to judge the cause of a patient's mental signs, and must be consulted, not only brings potential AIDS patients further into the workings of the medical system, it introduces them to still more (prescription) drugs to adjust mental states. Based on what? In the journal *Psychosomatics* (August, 1986, vol. 27, p. 562, James Dilly et al), there is a discussion of ethical and psychiatric issues involved in treating AIDS patients. The authors conclude, in one section, "In the case of AIDS or other terminal diseases . . . medical and legal scholars continue to debate whether suicide is a moral wrong and/or whether intervention by physicians or the police is warranted. No clear medical, moral, or legal consensus exists that suicide is always wrong in this group."

AIDS patients are being allowed to believe that their "illness" is invariably terminal, and in the case of dementia that, since the HIV virus is irreversibly affecting their brains, they may legitimately consider suicide.

The general movement of the medical establishment is to make the terminal AIDS diagnosis *earlier*, and if this trend continues, based on anecdotal reports from clinic administrators, soon patients who simply test positive for the HIV virus will be told, in so many words, "This condition is lethal."

One patient, recently diagnosed with AIDS in Los Angeles, left his doctor and began to try various unapproved treatments. Several months later, he returned to the doctor and told him, based on lab work, his blood tests were showing definite signs of improvement. He was feeling a great deal more energy.

His doctor said, "You're imagining you're getting better. You probably have AIDS dementia. The virus has gone to your brain."

Another patient's doctor suggested he get in touch with a physician in Holland, where euthanasia is practiced.

Diagnose a patient as having early dementia on the basis of a few vague symptoms and a virus which has not been proved to cause anything; prescribe new drugs for his mental state; give him the idea the condition is terminal, and that he is mentally incompetent; possibly suggest he consider suicide, or at least make it respectable. Is this coming to pass?

CHAPTER EIGHTEEN

AN INTERVIEW WITH DR. JOSEPH SONNABEND

Dr. Joseph Sonnabend spent ten years working at the British National Institute for Medical Research (their equivalent of our NIH). He is a member of the British Royal College of Physicians, has been Associate Professor of Medicine at the Mount Sinai Medical School in New York City. Since 1978, he has been treating patients in New York for sexually transmitted diseases and AIDS. For several years in the mid-1980s, he was the editor of the journal, *AIDS Research*.

That journal, now exclusively concentrating on HIV, was once the only true independent voice in AIDS research. Sonnabend was released from his position by the publisher when it became apparent that his approach to AIDS was in serious conflict with the more widely accepted HIV-view.

I spoke with him on March 25th, 1988.

Q: Where did the HIV hypothesis come from?

A: Several places. One of them involved a very sloppy analysis by the CDC of the first Los Angeles AIDS patients.

Q: From proposing that AIDS comes from a number of sources acting in concert, to proposing that AIDS is not a single disease-entity at all, seems a short step.

A: That's right.

Q: So if a patient comes in with pneumocystis, you could try to learn what produced the immuno-suppression that led to that pneumocystis – and once you learned that, there would be no reason to use the word AIDS. There would be no reason to go further and say there is something *else* that patient has called AIDS.

A: That's right. I would go along with that.

Q: In which case, the HIV thesis would seem to be operating as a diversion from the truth.

A: Yes. There is a history to this. There was such a hasty process – the worst thing that happened was the announcement in 1984 that HIV had been discovered to be the cause of AIDS. That did damage to the whole scientific endeavor.

There are social factors here, you know, in the whole presumption that every disease has a single agent. Some people want to believe that nothing we do in our lives, in our environments, is really unhealthy. That poverty is really not a bad thing, just a choice, and it doesn't make people sick. That sexual behavior and lifestyles are really harmless. The single-agent idea of disease, when believed across the board, at the expense of environmental factors, absolves people whose economic policies create ghettos and keep people poor. It's so easy to say that a virus came along and made people sick, not their living conditions. People who live a highly promiscuous lifestyle prefer to believe that the really lethal effects are external to that life, and are from a virus that comes along. Or in Africa, it's much easier to say that illness from the collapse of malaria-eradication programs or hunger is really due to HIV.

We're hung up on high-tech solutions. The one-agent theory is going to be attractive to researchers. All the funding went that way. It's also the attraction of the quick-fix, the quick cure.

The single-agent theory, in the case of AIDS, will have tremendous appeal for those political people who are promoting agendas based on what they call "family values." Or no sex outside of marriage. That sort of agenda.

There really is now such a thing as the AIDS-establishment. It is a group which receives virtually all the grant money, it sits on important boards (such as the fund raising organization, Americans for AIDS Research). There is definitely a group, and sadly, it's not the best talent.

Q: Did it ever seem to you that some researchers had malicious intent?

A: Toward who? People with AIDS?

Q: Yes.

A: I would find that hard to believe . . . that would be awful. It's possible that an individual here or there might, but a group . . . I think it's more likely that they have ego problems, they're stupid, they think nothing of pushing their own ideas as fact. It's a mixture of arrogance, egomania, and stupidity.

Q: It's obvious from talking with a number of scientists that there are people who have questions about HIV, but they won't open their mouths publicly because they're afraid of losing grant money or their jobs.

A: They're probably justified in feeling that.

Q: Is this something new, the pervasiveness of this fear?

A: No. Of course, with HIV, the *degree* to which that hypothesis closed all debate was monumental. I'm sure it's affected me.

In the beginning, when people were saying that HTLV-1[1] caused AIDS, that was patently absurd. Later on, when HTLV-1 was rejected, there was a claim made which supposedly explained *how* the mistake could have been made. It was that HTLV-1 was reacting similarly to HIV (in blood tests). But the French didn't find that to be so at all. So where were the researchers jumping up and down pointing out all this? They certainly weren't getting published.

Q: I've had people say to me, if HIV doesn't cause AIDS, why do so many scientists around the world say it does?

A: It's a selection process. The ones who agree HIV causes AIDS get their articles printed.

Q: But then people also like to maintain that if HIV were a mistake, some famous scientists would have spoken out publicly by now.

A: That's ridiculous. That's terrible. That's ascribing a quality to researchers that doesn't exist. One thing that's come out of all this AIDS business which I should have known already . . . you'd think that these researchers would have more respect for the truth, more social conscience. But these researchers are like anybody else. They fight for their jobs, they're intimidated, they don't stand up. They

---

[1] A virus purportedly connected with leukemia.

have the arrogance to think they're more interested in the truth than other people are.

In 1984 or 5, there was a science writer's workshop in New York. This was just after America had grown its first isolate of HIV, which looked exactly like the isolate the French had grown first. When the sequencing of these two isolates was done, they looked *too* much alike. They were virtually identical. This of course leads one to infer that the isolation of HIV here was done by simply growing the sample Montagnier and the French team had just sent us. That there was only *one* sample.

Well, during this workshop, I was standing out in the hall, speaking with a Nobel prize winner, an American, and I told him that we needed to tell these reporters about the identity of these two isolates of HIV, that there was something bad going on. And this man said, "Please don't do it. I wish you wouldn't." He's a self-righteous person who thinks he's the guardian of scientific propriety. You know, he's one of those who believes the public shouldn't see how filthy our operations are, that we'll sort it out for ourselves, we scientists. This is an elitist view.

Q: One claim for HIV as the cause of AIDS comes from the fact that it kills human T-cells in the lab.

A: The fact that a virus can kill a cell in vitro has nothing to do with what it does in the human body. There are any number of viruses that will kill human cells in vitro very efficiently. But you can drink them, by the gallon, and nothing will happen. At any rate, HIV doesn't reliably kill cells in vitro.

You know, one of the papers we published in *AIDS Research* showed that, from the blood of 60 or 70 AIDS patients, after analysis by three different well-known labs, there wasn't a sign of HTLV-1 in any of that blood. This was at the period when the theory was that HTLV-1 was the cause of AIDS. The author sent that paper around to the usual journals, and they all turned it down. This is part of the informal stranglehold on AIDS research that exists. The paper was a very angry piece about the stupidity of HTLV-1. I published it in *AIDS Research* and I toned the language down. And I regret now that I did tone it down.

So there may very well be people who now question HIV. But they aren't getting a scientific forum.

Q: There are supposedly several different AIDS viruses all causing this unique thing called AIDS.

A: I'm amazed that people haven't pointed out the stupidity of that idea. Here we have HIV-1 and HIV-2. These two *separate* viruses, not strains of each other. The variance between them is considerable. Now they're said to be causing the same new disease-entity, AIDS. These two viruses would have had to evolve independently over untold amounts of time to arrive, by chance, at the same moment, with both just happening to cause the same thing. The odds against that are virtually impossible.

Q: You did early research on interferon in AIDS patients, which showed they had persistent, elevated levels. Why are some researchers doing studies in which they give AIDS patients *more* interferon? It's immunosuppressive, isn't it?

A: Definitely. No good is coming of it. I asked an interferon researcher how they could continue to give AIDS patients this when it had such clear immunosuppressive properties. He said well, the drug companies had such huge unsold stocks of recombinant interferon – anything that would make the annual shareholder meeting a happy event . . . There is a tremendous incompetence along with this. There are people, you know, who take tremendous pride in the AZT trials. They think they were wonderful. That trial was so wrong, so badly done. It's terrible.

AIDS has become an international business, an industry. It could be assessed at billions of dollars.

Q: A certain amount of responsibility has to be laid at the door of doctors who prescribed anything from poppers, by the ton, to God knows what for their gay patients.

A: Oh yes. I know that among some doctors who developed large clienteles of gay patients, there was a great reluctance to make judgments about the so-called lifestyle. There was a kind of philosophy that you couldn't change behavior. I fell into that myself, but after a year or so, I shed it. I mean, I saw young men who should have been so healthy, and here they'd had two bouts of hepatitis, syphilis,

and so on. It was a terrible thing. So I really didn't have a problem
starting to tell people about the risks they were running. And I didn't
turn any of my patients off.

PART TWO

LAMBS OF THE MEDIA AND POLITICAL SCAPEGOATS

CHAPTER NINETEEN

OFFICIAL, BIZARRE DEFINITIONS OF AIDS

Most of the several hundred scientists I spoke with had little to contribute to the question of whether HIV causes human disease, or immune-suppression, or anything else; simply because they accept without question that, if other medical authorities say HIV is the culprit, that must be true.

I was quite surprised to find this out. These medical people did not *defend* the choice of HIV as the most virulent thing to come along since automobiles, they simply said in essence, "So many researchers agree that HIV is the cause of AIDS, it must be."

When I raised the question of whether AIDS itself was one coherent entity, or just a collection of symptoms and separate diseases, I was met with even *less* considered thinking. To 99% of these people, the existence of a Central Reality called AIDS was a completely foregone conclusion. If I was so bold, on occasion, to ask for proof, for journal citations, I suddenly found myself up against defensive attitudes. But no proof.

Predictable, I suppose.

If AIDS was never proved to stem from one virus; if its main symptoms, pneumocystis and Kaposi, show no particular tie to that virus, then what are we left with?

Several very broad definitions of AIDS are used around the world. It is interesting to look at them. They clearly have the effect of rounding up all sorts of diverse symptoms which doctors, in their wildest dreams, wouldn't ordinarily think of lumping together.

First, there is the current CDC definition, used in the U.S. and parts of Africa. It was announced in August-September of 1987, printed in the *Journal of the American Medical Association* on September 4, 1987, and is reprinted in full in Appendix 3 of this book.

A document for the ages, it lists about 25 separate diseases/infections and several categories of diseases. Any single disease or category is sufficient for a diagnosis of AIDS under most conditions.

A very strange thing is, after four years of research to find a virus which supposedly causes AIDS, this CDC definition allows for diagnoses of AIDS which don't require positive blood tests for HIV.

There are, in fact, now three doors through which one can walk into a diagnosis of AIDS. At one door, an unknown or uncertain HIV test result is no barrier. At another entrance, a *negative* HIV test, likewise, is no obstacle.

Is the CDC admitting that HIV has little to do with AIDS? Not publicly, that's certain. Reading through the long document, one comes on a truly amazing statement (p. 1149, *JAMA*, Sept. 4, 1987): "Approximately one third of AIDS patients in the United States have been from New York City and San Francisco, where, since 1985, less than 7% have been reported (to the CDC) with HIV-antibody test results, compared with greater than 60% in other areas."

How could this be? This is saying that doctors simply haven't bothered giving the HIV blood-test to their patients; or if they have, they haven't forwarded the results to the CDC.

I spoke with several people at the CDC, and came away with confusion as the only answer. One spokesperson said she was sure you could always have been diagnosed with AIDS, even though you didn't have a positive HIV test. The other spokesperson said, as far as he was concerned, a positive HIV test has always been necessary, ever since the HIV test was developed in 1985. A third source, a statistician, told me the problem of reporting no HIV test results was not the CDC's, it stemmed from the health authorities in New York and California; possibly the reason for the delinquency was a lack of faith in the accuracy of the tests.

Regardless, the fact is, for the last three years, the overwhelming number of AIDS cases in the U.S. have been recorded by the CDC with no knowledge of whether or not the patients have tested positive for the HIV virus.

This throws into question its entire tally of AIDS cases.

The September, 1987, definition also, in essence, puts the whole matter of AIDS diagnosis back to square one. In the early 80s, physicians were looking at diseases like pneumocystis and wondering what had caused the underlying immunosuppression. A research effort was mounted which resulted in the announcement of the cause: HIV. Regardless of the fact that the announcement was based on no solid proof, it became the central "discovery" of the AIDS research establishment. At that point, physicians, faced with infections and diseases that seemed to be related to AIDS, blood-tested their patients for the presence of HIV. Now, that test is no longer required to read positive. Now, the physician, looking at a case of, say, pneumocystis, can just *assume* this is AIDS. As shaky as HIV-associated AIDS always was, this new permissiveness is even more absurd. Out of thin air, it says, "Assume all these infections/diseases are AIDS."

No proof. Instead, a word game, a piece of flim-flam. Simply associate the word AIDS with a host of infections previously known as separate entities.

I won't try to list these "AIDS-related" diseases and infections in the definition. You can read the considerable list, in full glory, in Appendix 3. I'll only point out that there is a new category which makes it possible for any person under the sun to now be diagnosed as having AIDS. The category is: "And other bacterial infections."

Those physicians I have told about this definition (they hadn't seen it) were flabbergasted.

One doctor commented, "The worst part is, with all the hysteria about AIDS, diagnoses will be even looser than the definition. Whatever latitude the definition now allows, some doctors will be slapping on AIDS labels at the drop of a hat. With this wasting-syndrome business, for example, some doctors won't really do the tests to see whether the cause of the weight loss comes from some unusual parasites . . . they'll just call it AIDS."

The Western Journal of Medicine, (December 1987, p. 695) reports that international AIDS cases are now based on two or possibly three different definitions, a muddled proposition. The so-called Bangui/WHO definition at least makes a note that severe malnutrition should rule out a diagnosis of AIDS. But it doesn't attempt to spell out how a doctor is really going to draw the line, when he sees the so-called major African AIDS symptoms – weight loss, diarrhea, and fever – and tries to figure out what part of that is being caused by germs or chemicals, and what part by lingering chronic long-term malnutrition.

Then there is the CDC definition of AIDS I have just discussed. That is also being used as a criterion in some African areas, with its category, "other bacterial infections," any one of which can add up to a straight-out label of AIDS. The third possibility is the Swedish-Tanzanian proposed definition (*Lancet*, October 24, 1987), in which severe malnutrition is not specifically stressed as non-AIDS and otherwise pretty much mirrors the Bangui definition.

Generally, on the international scene, rampant malnutrition and tropical disease, causing immune-suppression, can easily be called AIDS. All immune-suppression leads to opportunistic infections, and this is the pattern which, in Johnny-come-lately fashion, has now been defined as AIDS.

In fact, authors Peter Piot and Robert Colebunders, writing for the World Health Organization in the *Western Journal of Medicine* (December, 1987), make the following astonishing remark: "The major changes in the case definition (of AIDS) are the inclusion of . . . AIDS patients whose indicator diseases are diagnosed presumptively (without specific lab tests), *and the elimination of the requirement of the absence of other causes of immunodeficiency*." (Emphasis added.)

That last is the killer. No longer will it be necessary to make sure the potential AIDS patient isn't suffering from some other non-AIDS immunodeficiency, before slapping on a diagnosis.

Now any immune depressed condition is all right to lump under AIDS. All those pneumocystis patients who were developing the pneumonia because they had leukemia and were being given immunotoxic drugs? AIDS. All those people with hypogammaglobulinemia[1] , who weren't producing antibodies to *anything*? Who were sprouting opportunistic infections like crazy? AIDS.

---

[1] A shortage of gammaglobulin, which contains many antibodies.

The list, believe me, is very long. There are other older medical conditions which can closely resemble what is called AIDS: Hashimoto's Disease, Severe Combined Immunodeficiency (SCID), Di George Syndrome. Di George can give rise to pneumocystis, candidiasis, CMV, and atypical mycobacteria – all of which are indicator diseases for AIDS by the latest definitions.

To say nothing of the immunosuppressive effects of drugs, drugs, and more drugs, medical and recreational. And starvation.

In the same issue of the *Western Journal of Medicine*, a new category is defined for us: it is called "early HIV disease." Supposedly, this can occur one week after contacting HIV, before a blood test would even register antibodies to the virus.

"Several studies," authors Piot and Colebunders write, "have now described the clinical manifestations of early HIV disease. Fever, lymphadenopathy (infected glands), night sweating, headache and cough were all significantly associated with seroconversion (becoming antibody-positive to HIV). One third to one half of patients with seroconversion report at least one of these symptoms."

Where does one start with this? First, a table of statistics is offered, and as far as I can tell, the two studies it illustrates involved a grand total of 62 patients. To define a new illness.

Next, headache or cough are enough to rank one as having "early HIV disease."

The existence of this new illness is demonstrated because *one-third to one-half of the patients interviewed had at least one listed symptom*. A headache? A cough?

Here is one more little bit of assumed novelty, a new phase for AIDS, one more opportunity to target a patient with the word AIDS. We may next hear that early AIDS can be cured with a Chericol and soda and two Excedrin.

Finally, a note on one of the infections now sufficient for a diagnosis of AIDS. *JAMA*, Dec. 11, 1987, reports on the largest outbreak of salmonellosis in US history: between 168,000 and 197,000 people. Two interesting facts. The salmonella was resistant to antibiotics, and its source was a pasteurized milk plant. Bad milk plus overprescription of antibiotics equal AIDS?

The CDC uses a ploy to defend its definition of AIDS: In attempting to carry out surveillance on the "spreading of AIDS cases," it must allow for the widest possible definitions to be used, so that few cases escape the net; one, naturally, would not expect a physician with a single patient to apply such lax requirements in coming to a conclusion the patient had AIDS.

Unfortunately, in this day and age, people are not making a careful distinction, in practice, between the CDC definition and the practicing of good medicine. The public spotlight is shining so hard on AIDS that any sort of diagnosis – surveillance, clinical – whatever, is going to function as a death sentence.

Can you see an employee saying to his boss, "My doctor told me I had a *surveillance* case of AIDS. It isn't exactly the same as a *real* case, but he has to report it, you see. It's nothing to worry about . . ."

It doesn't take a genius to figure out the effect of these various definitions of AIDS. By taking major symptoms of malnutrition, for example – fever, wasting-away, and diarrhea – and calling them AIDS, the numbers of reported cases will grow. By placing under a single AIDS umbrella numerous infections and diseases, the numbers of reported cases will grow. By eliminating the need for even a positive HIV blood test, the numbers of cases will grow.

The greater the number of reported cases, the greater the apparent threat to public health all over the world. Ultimately this will reflect in treatment, by drugs and vaccines. Pharmaceutical profits will soar.

Several months ago, a Doctor Herbert Ratner of Oak Park, Illinois, told me the following story: Back in 1954-5, when he was public health officer for Oak Park, just before the introduction of the first polio vaccine, the National Foundation for Infantile Paralysis was paying physicians $25 for every reported diagnosis of paralytic polio. So Ratner said, "A patient would walk into the doctor's office with a limp from an accident. He'd say he had a fever a few days ago . . . and guess what the diagnosis would be?"

Paralytic polio. Ratner also stated it was well-known paralytic polio cured itself 50% of the time within sixty days. After the Salk vaccine was introduced, the definition of polio was changed. Now, in order to have paralytic polio, you had to have it *longer* than sixty days.

Quite a shell-game, if true. First, inflate case statistics by offering to pay for reported diagnoses of the disease; then, after the vaccine is introduced, change the definition so that it will look like numbers of cases plummeted. Of course, people don't believe such devious strategies really go on in the pristine world of medicine. But look what is happening with AIDS now. We are in the definition-expanding phase. Once the AIDS-vaccine arrives with the cavalry, some bright researcher might make a breakthrough and discover that AIDS is really much more *specific* in its symptoms than previously thought. This researcher will be pleasantly shocked to find his work hailed and broadcast instantly and accepted, not only by the public, but practitioners of medicine.

1) The definition of a disease expands. Case numbers swell.

2) Drugs/vaccines are introduced.

3) The definition contracts. Case numbers reduce.

Could it happen? Yes.

Why hasn't the mainstream media covered this definitional aspect of AIDS?

CHAPTER TWENTY

MEDIA AND THE AIDS PARTY-LINE

Once there was a war on cancer, an epic struggle carried on at NIH during the 1970s. Richard Nixon was advised to support public health, because Ted Kennedy was likely to run against him in the 1972 election. Nixon declared the war, and scientists were drafted into the ranks and sent out to do battle.

Two factions developed; one, rather secretive for a time, believed that cancer was caused by substances generated out of our industrial society. The other faction, eventually led by Robert Gallo, looked for viruses. In the end, no one won. Gallo discovered two human leukemia viruses, which today are written about with much more circumspection than in the early triumphant days of their unearthing. Meanwhile, the environmentalists let the issue get so out of hand it took hundreds of pages just to list the environmental compounds which might cause cancer and/or cell-mutation.

Arguments like this have raged before. Smallpox, which we take to be a viral illness entirely preventable by inoculation, has been accused of daring to decline in late nineteenth-century England because of improvement in sanitation alone.

Epidemics of cholera in Africa in the late 1970s were treated widely with antibiotics. But reports are that the best management came in Zaire, where antibiotics were underplayed, and the emphasis was put on improving sanitation and handing out salt-sugar packets which, mixed with water, reversed the terrible dehydration cholera brings on.

With AIDS, the media have chosen not to become embroiled in the question of causation. Media get their information from press people who work at universities and public health agencies, and who are fed HIV-dogma like popcorn.

If you are a reporter and call research institutions looking for information, you are shunted to PR folks who, though earnest enough, are paid not to think on their own.

They relay information given to them from department heads of various labs where research is going on.

They also screen out requests for information which are embarrassing. A number of reporters, for example, have called the National Cancer Institute, wanting to speak with Robert Gallo about his rock-solid conviction that HIV causes AIDS. He has become notorious for refusing to discuss this question, especially if the name of his current nemesis, Peter Duesberg, is mentioned.

Duesberg is finally, at this late date, getting some of the press he deserves, but for the first seven years of AIDS, no one who forwarded a non-viral or (after 1984) a non-HIV cause for AIDS was given prime space.

Why? Because the official line daily newspapers print comes down from NIH and CDC. That's just the way things run (with notable exceptions, like Nick Regush at the *Montreal Gazette*, John Crewdson at the *Chicago Tribune*, and Terry Krieger and Dr. Cesar Caceres, who have contributed to the *Wall St. Journal*).

Writers for dailies don't get paid to do research in bio-med libraries, to *put together* pieces of information they actually dig up on their own from medical literature or human sources. Therefore, federal health agencies are always going to sound right and authoritative to reporters.

Also, for a writer, not pleasing an editor, going outside traditional sources of info could lead to excessive wonderment on the editor's part about whether to trust said writer. Is said writer deserting the time-honored grove of anonymity, in which Reasonable Authority has the final word? Is said writer beginning to speak for himself based on his own research? Is said writer, fool that he is, about to risk his paycheck looking for unknown facts on a highly controversial story? Is he trying to become an authority without the proper credentials? Who said this character could shoot off his mouth without a medical degree?

Said daily staff writer knows all these questions drift in the ether like inactivated germs which, after enough wrong moves on his part, could be triggered and bring about his firing.

There is a degree of sheer politeness and good form involved here too. An obvious media assumption is: Things Are Generally All Right.

A writer knows how close he is getting to questioning the basic sense of an issue, he knows when he is about to turn over the cart and everything in it and say some issue or another is a *con*.

This is breaking the central rule: Things are Generally All Right. This is like walking into a Washington cocktail party with soup all over your suit.

On a story like AIDS, very quickly you begin to realize you're going to contradict a lot of conventional wisdom, not just in a single aspect, but in every aspect. You're going to point out that the whole research program, as vast as it is coming to be, as many stars in relevant fields as it is beginning to employ, is on a crash course to Nowhere.

If you work on staff for a major daily paper, you are going to steer clear of this recognition. It's self-damaging if you act on it.

Investigative reporting costs money. On a story of any proportion, there are so many layers, so many people to locate, that you'll go broke as a writer unless someone is backing you up with a decent wage for months on end. During which time, nothing gets published.

Editors, besides bowing to the basic rule of Things Being All Right, know they can't justify spending money on a story which takes a great deal of time. They'll do a few of them, but they'll pick their shots. Science is almost never one of those shots. It's too wrapped up in mists at the top of the federal towers, where supposedly only a few highly polished medical domes know what's really what.

So here with AIDS, media reluctance and mass hypnosis meet. The men in the white coats are kings. They scoot in polished labs and issue proclamations now and then, and the populace listens through the media and pays obligatory homage.

All the more reason to be wary of death sentences handed out by white coats. The power, for some patients is close to ultimate. If a person will jump off a building because he tested positive for HIV, you know something is going on. Something in part called cultural hypnotism because, admit it, that hysterical person hadn't the slightest idea whether his disease, if any, was going to be fatal or not. He was operating on pure faith.

There are books which have been written about the ownership of media, about the tastes and prejudices and agendas of the people who actually own newspapers and television stations. It's not the purpose of this book to do an excavation on that subject; but it does occur to me that maybe there was a time when these owners had to exercise more day-to-day control, just to make sure their attitudes were being reflected in the output of their employees.

But now there is a tendency for things to run smoothly all by themselves. Writers for major papers and TV stations are in no need of lecture, correction, and navigation. Without prodding, most turn out what, in the eyes of their betters, should be turned out. They behave well at the cocktail party.

It's easy to miss the cumulative effect of many, many people "correctly" building up an issue like AIDS over seven or eight years. The juggernaut thus created is very hard to turn around.

First there is the fact that epidemics are perfect events for media work. We have the invisible killer. It moves silently, unpredictably, without tipping its hand.

We meet victims.

We get a constant barrage of new scientific information, breakthroughs. This gives readers the impression they're peering over the shoulders of the best minds of our time, delving into the mysteries of the gene, the virus, the core-essence of human life.

We get terror. It might be me. I might be the next person to be sneezed on by a junky, even though I know I can't get the virus from sneezes. But maybe I can. That lab worker stuck her hand on a needle. That's all it took. And then some AIDS victim *bled* all over the cop who shot him with a stun gun in LA. I wonder if the cop's suing. My girlfriend and I . . . we've only been living together for four years. She could have picked up the virus when she was in Baltimore. Who was that scuzzball she used to go out with?

It's called whipsawing, *from pillar to post.*

One newspaper in the U.S. has managed to avoid all this baloney, and it's worth mentioning. The *New York Native* is small. Partly because it had no chance of influencing the AIDS issue by pretending to be the *New York Times*, partly because publisher Chuck Ortleb started it on $500 (which tells you it can't outfit bureaus abroad and drag in every detail of AIDS from around the world), and partly because of Ortleb's interest in making a good kind of trouble, this paper has kept alive the AIDS issue in New York as no other media outlet has.

The approach has been simple: attack. In this, the *Native* harkens back to what we fondly like to call (did it ever really exist?) the muck-raking tradition in American journalism.

The *Native* has approached scientific issues surrounding AIDS with none of usual get-a-few-statements-from-both-sides pap. They've put people on to AZT, for example, with the purpose of *actually deciding the issue.* How dangerous is the drug? How were the original studies on it done? They've put Peter Duesberg on the cover, carrying on the only intelligent dissenting conversation in America concerning HIV and its non-role in AIDS.

They've pointed out that the New York City Health Department buried the question of whether African Swine Fever might be implicated in AIDS. They've helped bring the black community of New York into the issue, by printing on their front page, a short sketch of the infamous Tuskegee *Syphilis Study* (1932-72), in which four hundred poor black sharecroppers were observed, without treatment, were kept from *getting* treatment, unto death by syphilis, for purposes of scientific study. The experiment was run by CDC and U.S. Public Health Service officials. With some current researchers raising the question of a possible syphilis-AIDS connection, the *Native* simply asked, is this connection being ignored, is malignant neglect the order of the day, is AIDS in New York a continuation of the Tuskegee Syphilis Study?

Ortleb printed a letter on his front cover, an open letter to Mayor Koch, replete with assurances that *everyone knows* the good Mayor wouldn't purposely condone a continuation of the Tuskegee

Study in New York City, but would His Honor please get on it and find out why the hell the New York City Health Dept. is dragging its heels looking into an AIDS-syphilis link?

This may not be the sober and stolid way to present issues, but in a city that leads the world in AIDS, the paper operates out of a battlefront mentality which blasts issues home. They are actually trying to solve the AIDS mystery, not report on it. They know how to apply heat, and it's a different thing to see, because even the alternative newspapers in America seem to be losing their grip on how to do that. Most of them are trying to become bureaucracies.

Our big-city papers fulfill the function of gathering information of great diversity, but the feeling in all media is that a frame is built around news – which forestalls public debate and action.

With AIDS, media move away from judging the scientific issues, which, after all, are the heart of solving the disease. Or should be. We get almost nothing questioning the *science*. We get nothing about university researchers who are rankling under the collar because they can't get a dime to do viral research unless they write *I Believe In HIV* at the top of their application forms. We get nothing about issues which might affect curing AIDS.

If we rely on the fact that NIH science itself will resolve AIDS, it's pretty easy to dismiss the media doldrum as inconsequential. But several factors within the scientific community mitigate against a resolution of AIDS and here again, major dailies (to say nothing of TV news) hide their heads in the sand.

I think a few of the major dailies should do a survey, off the record, among university and health-agency scientists around the U.S., and ask them if they feel political matters have become prominent in: obtaining grants to do research on AIDS, getting AIDS articles published in journals. Part of the definition of "political," of course, is *having* to assume HIV causes AIDS.

There is an ordinary fact of life in scientific circles called peer review. AMA executives like to sing its praises. Its most manic proponents claim it is responsible for most of science's advances. What it amounts to is simply this: in determining what articles are printed in technical journals, in deciding what grant applications are funded, scientists judge their fellows. No outsiders allowed.

By outsiders are meant civilians who lack credentialed technical expertise. At first glance, this seems right. After all, who are we to know the value of a grant-project, its feasibility?

However, the point is, civilians have a right to be interested in the direction science is taking, what priorities are being emphasized, what risks are being ignored. These issues are mostly buried in the minds of scientists themselves. The above-mentioned Tuskegee Syphilis Study is a prime and extreme example of what can happen when peer review is the total order of the day. See James Jones' excellent *Bad Blood* (Macmillan, 1981) for a thorough treatment of the Tuskegee Study.

For 40 years, until reporters blew the whistle, medical bureaucrats perpetuated, and reaffirmed periodically with funding, a project that hid the fact that 400 black men in Alabama had syphilis. The reason for the project? Observing human syphilis in its late stages – until these men's symptoms spread all the way to death.

Even after penicillin had become the drug of choice in the U.S., around 1950, a conscious decision was made to withhold medication from the 400 men. Of course, their children and wives never found out what was going on either. As the men died, one by one, they were autopsied and their diseased parts were sent to NIH for analysis.

Local doctors in Macon County were all too eager, when approached, to cooperate with the medical bureaucrats in Washington, who needed "field professionals" to assure that, if the "experimental subjects" went to doctors on their own, they wouldn't be given penicillin for any reason, because that would affect the natural course of their disease. Local physicians who went along with the project felt they were part of something important, a large purpose. Not one of them asked why the sharecroppers would not be treated or told they had syphilis.

As far as the subjects of the experiments themselves were concerned, they believed they were simply being treated for ill-health. The pink pills handed out during their physical examinations were probably aspirin. Nothing stronger.

Obviously, to be carried out, the Tuskegee Study required the cooperation of many scientific bureaucrats. Also obviously, untrained citizens, had they been sitting on review boards as requests for continued funding came up (and how many times do you think that was, over a *forty-year period*) – these citizens would have raised questions. They would have asked about messy matters like murder. The hypnotic spell created by the wand of Science would have been shattered.

Never has any person been fined or prosecuted for his role in the Tuskegee Study.

With AIDS, no newspaper probes the fact that peer review has, politically, established HIV as the starting point for all research, has ruled out other research, no matter how promising, where HIV is not the basis.

A virologist at a southern California university said, when I asked him about HIV as the cause of AIDS: "There are those of us who stand back a little from the political fray . . . and see that they really haven't proved HIV causes AIDS. Medical faddism isn't new, you know. The Swedes, in 1911, did important research on polio, but the substance of their work was ignored here until 1950, because research in America had been heading along a different channel."

This was off the record.

At another southern California university, several virologists were read the latest CDC definition of AIDS. When they realized that a positive HIV test was no longer needed for a diagnosis, they practically fell off their chairs. One of them was heard to splutter, "That's . . . illegal!" But, of course, no one would go on the record with that reaction, or any reaction. In fact, one of the researchers emphasized his neutrality by remarking, "Are you crazy? Do you think I'm going to stick my neck out on *this* business?"

Professionals frightened for their jobs, their grant monies. They will not take a contrary or critical position on AIDS. A good part of that fear stems from the tacit threat that peer review, among their own conservative kind, will shut them down, leave them without grants, publishable articles, and ultimately jobs.

Big daily newspapers will present as fact that a diagnosis of HIV-positive is nearly tantamount to future death – an assertion entirely unsupported by broad-spectrum studies – but they don't dare suggest that, below the surface of academia, there is a lot of resentment about the way AIDS research is being managed. *That* they call unsubstantiated rumor.

We've also been led to believe that *more funds* is the only controversial issue. Media play is now being given to that analysis. The truth is, more money thrown down the same hole that produced HIV and AZT, etc., is questionable money. Very questionable. But to say that more than just a lack of money is rotten in Denmark violates the cardinal rule: Things Are Basically All Right. It is impolite to suggest that structural supports are rotten, that problems are endemic, that AIDS research is a swimming mess and will stay that way.

If a major media outlet decided to pursue AIDS contradictions and scandals with a mean, day-after-day approach, exposing every aspect, not relenting, giving front-page coverage and headlines often enough to keep the public in a mild frenzy, then you might see upper management step in, you might see media-ownership make a move to put the squash on proceedings, because then the natives would have gotten out of hand with an issue which is too sensitive.

When NIH turned the corner into the 1980s, it was sailing with a broken mast. Its program on cancer had been a flop compared with expectations generated in the professional community and in the public mind. Then AIDS arrived. NIH determined that Robert Gallo, one of those men who had worked with so-called cancer viruses, the new class called retroviruses, would get the nod on pursuing the search for an AIDS germ. The technology was in place. The equipment was there. It was high-tech.

Gallo has proved to be adept at controlling the direction of research. He has minimized, with help, the number of causation-scenarios which will be entertained. More than any other American researcher, he has belittled environmental factors, belittled the non-HIV models of AIDS. Zombie-like, the press has cooperated.

When newspapers do report something that lies under the surface, it usually dies after a day or two.

For example, on October 22nd, 1987, the makings of a major scandal broke in the *New York Times*.

The New York City Health Dept. challenged AIDS death-statistics released by the CDC. Seems that instead of 31% of AIDS deaths in NYC resulting from IV drug use, a much larger 53% was the correct figure.

What this meant was, diagnosed AIDS in NY was more IV-drug than gay. The CDC had been saying 55% of all AIDS deaths in the city were male gays. The New York City Health Dept. said no, that figure should be 38%.

You would be hard pressed to dig up any more info on this story. It died. No scandal erupted. No major conflict emerged at the CDC.

It actually was the tail end of detective work done two years earlier by Terry Krieger and Dr. Cesar Caceres (*Wall St. Journal*, October 24, 1985), and still earlier by John Lauritsen (*Philadelphia Gay News*, Feb. 14,1985).

Although the two 1985 pieces were a bit different from each other, their message was essentially the same: AIDS is a drug-related phenomenon, almost across the board. Throw out the risk-groups and just look into the backgrounds of those diagnosed with AIDS and you will, in the overwhelming majority of cases, find drug abuse.

Since these stories made an obvious kind of sense, they were ignored.

Researchers had been explaining IV drug use as AIDS-related by invoking dirty, shared needles as the cause. That gave them a scenario for viral transmission, which was what they were looking for. And in the case of homosexual sex, they cited semen to blood transmission in anal intercourse as the probable route of HIV transmission.

But they overlooked and ignored another factor. Drugs. The drugs the IV users were shooting up every day and the immunosuppressive effect of that, which fact to any ordinary observer would hang like a fifty-foot neon sign in the air.

Furthermore, the CDC, in its AIDS statistics, had invented the IV drug-user category for heterosexuals only. Those gay men who also shot drugs were put in the gay/bisexual category, because it was *assumed* that gay sex was the way they had contracted AIDS.

Turned out, reported Krieger and Caceres, "If we add the 1,163 homosexual and bisexual IV drug users to the 2,342 exclusively heterosexual IV drug users, we find at least 25% of AIDS patients have been intravenous drug users."

Krieger and Caceres, then invoking several CDC surveys of AIDS patients, projected that at least 54% of AIDS patients had been *oral* drug abusers. 54 plus 25 equals 79. ". . . we find that at least 79% of AIDS patients have been drug abusers."

Let me tell you, the joy of being able to detect one virus in 79% of patients with a new disease would be cause for strutting in the halls of NIH.

But to discover that 79% of all those diagnosed with AIDS are quite possibly drug abusers makes no news. It falls flat. Well, there is no novel drug that can be manufactured and prescribed and sold to eradicate all drug use. Although as I write this, I'm sure somewhere in the world, a researcher is trying to invent just such a medication, and will be more than eager to overlook its undoubted hazardous side effects.

As of October, 1987, IV drug use was holding firm at 24% of all AIDS cases. In addition to that, the CDC reports that, of the blacks who have been diagnosed with AIDS, 42% have used IV drugs; in the Hispanic community, the percentage of IV drug users is also 42%. The coincidence of 42% makes one think these figures are estimates, but if they are close to the truth at all, they too reveal a major overlooked factor in AIDS. If we accept the Krieger-Caceres projection that 54% of AIDS patients are oral drug-abusers – or any figure *remotely* resembling that – we could be talking about 90+% of black and Hispanic AIDS patients abusing some form of drugs.

Of course, people have been using drugs for centuries. But not in these combinations, and not with these adulterants. More important, some heavy drug abusers *have*, historically, died of immunosuppression-plus-opportunistic-infections, the so-called AIDS pattern. It isn't new. They have developed wasting syndromes, pneumonias, rampant viral and bacterial infections which have killed them.

The Krieger and Caceres story appeared in the *Wall St. Journal* and promptly died. It became an interesting curio, nothing more.

CHAPTER TWENTY-ONE

INSTEAD OF THE EVENING NEWS

Suppose your TV set began telling you something important: that not one study of consequence had been done which tracked the changing health of those who *cut out damaging immunosuppressive factors from their lives*. But that story is too complicated for TV, and worse yet, it bites a hole in the rule: Things Are Basically All Right. You might conclude, if medical researchers aren't punching up better health by studying people who try to change detrimental habits, what the hell *are* they doing?

Suppose, since your TV set is already fixated on "human interest" stories, it began telling you about numbers of people who have been misdiagnosed as having AIDS. This must be happening all over the world.

A hit and miss scan of AIDS literature quickly turns up a few recorded examples.

Raymond Smego describes a case in "Secondary Syphilis Masquerading as AIDS in a Young Gay Male," (*North Carolina Medical Journal*, vol. 45, 1984, p. 253-4). Smego writes, "(The patient's presentation of) constitutional complaints, diffuse lymph node enlargement, and widespread skin lesions was mistakenly attributed to AIDS by both the patient and the medical staff upon admission. Indeed, many of these features were compatible with either the AIDS-related complex, which may represent a prodrome to the development of full-blown AIDS, or with disseminated KS (Kaposi's sarcoma)." The eventual conclusion, though, was that this patient had syphilis.

But once a disease gets rolling – and I mean in Washington, not in populations – you leave common sense behind.

RA Berg, in the July, 1986, *Southern Medical Journal*, describes an error in AIDS diagnosis: "A 29-year-old male Haitian refugee had generalized lymphadenopathy, weight loss, bilateral lung infiltrates,

AIDS INC.

diagnosed by transbronchial lung biopsy as tuberculosis. He had previously been labeled as having 'pre-AIDS' which led to multiple suicide attempts. Four months later, cyanosis and gangrene of both lower extremities necessitated amputation, which revealed vasculitis." *That* was the diagnosis, for which he *hadn't* been treated. Not AIDS.

Dr. Harry Hollander, of the Adult Immunodeficiency Clinic, at the University of California at San Francisco, summarized, in a 1986 study, 80 consecutive physician-referred patients he saw, who had been diagnosed "with AIDS-related illnesses." Eight of them turned out to be, as he called it, *pseudo-AIDS*. They actually had other medical illnesses, treatment of which was being derailed by the false diagnosis.

Here is one story from the eight: "The patient, a 20-year-old man, was referred by a physician-relative for concern of lymphadenopathy syndrome (infected glands). He is a physical laborer at a winery who complained of ten days of pain and fatigue beneath his right arm. His family assumed that he practiced a homosexual lifestyle because he lived with male companions, and therefore he was referred . . . The history showed recent heavy lifting at work that preceded the onset of pain. He said he had not engaged in homosexual activities or other activities known to be risk factors for AIDS. On examination there was only tenderness of the short head of the right biceps with a resolving ecchymosis overlying the mid-biceps. No adenopathy was appreciated. Results of a complete blood count and sedimentation rate were within normal limits . . ."

In other words, the proper diagnosis was muscle-strain.

Too many of these misdiagnoses might shake public confidence. In what, though? An AIDS research establishment which has yet to make a single right move?

In a recent issue of *Family Practice News* (December 15-31, 1987), Dr. Luc Montagnier, co-discoverer of the HIV virus, and Jonathan Mann, WHO spokesman for AIDS, both debunked the green monkey theory of AIDS' origin. The *Family Practice* article was covering an AIDS-in-Africa conference in Naples. Montagnier said some very weak arguments had been forwarded to put AIDS' origination in Africa and characterized the emergence of AIDS viruses as "a continuing mystery." Jonathan Mann told the conference, "The more information that emerges, the less we know about where this virus came from, how long it has been in the world, and how it grew to become the problem it is today."

Why hasn't this story moved from *Family Practice* to section one of major American newspapers? Why hasn't it been given a good kick on to the evening news?

Basically, because the press representatives at NIH and CDC haven't told American reporters that the story is true, that it has the official seal of approval from their scientists.

Robert Gallo and Max Essex, two of our highest-ranking AIDS researchers, still believe that AIDS originated in Africa, despite the fact that Essex recently retracted key research which had pointed to an African-monkey origin of an HIV-type virus.

So, for American reporters, the debunking of the African green monkey theory by one of HIV's discoverers is just a European opinion.

One night, instead of the evening news, I propose airing a fantasy, a fable told by a voice like Rather, Cronkite, or perhaps, better yet, Leonard Bernstein. A narration to an on-screen cartoon:

Boys and girls, forthwith the story of the suicide-gene.

In several big cities across America, simultaneously seventeen carpenters have committed suicide. This takes awhile to discover, of course. But computers, digesting facts of police inquiries all over the country bring this odd fact up. And, of course, it *is* an odd fact. Why should this happen? No one can answer that.

But right away a search commences for the cause. One enterprising researcher, Doctor X, has a pet theory. He's nursed this for years, has written articles about it, has garnered grant monies, has headed up investigative teams. The teams, though, don't actually go out into the field and paw over crimes, they study human genes in a lab in Maryland.

Doctor X believes that there is a gene in the human which controls the act of suicide. This gene can be switched on or switched off, but when it is ON, the owner of the gene eventually commits suicide. The suicide gene is hard to trigger, but when some unknown factor does it, there is no turning back. That's the basic reason for violence in the world, always has been.

All the hogwash about upbringing, poverty, drug addiction, abusive fathers, character flaws, juvenile jails, starvation – all this is incidental to the suicide gene. Without the gene being switched on, nothing happens.

Doctor X is overjoyed about these carpenters because it gives him a clear field for research.

Now suppose (and I'm not here trying to mimic what has actually been done in the field of human genetics) Doctor X has mapped out seven genes and claims to know what human functions they invariably regulate. Many journal articles argue against these "discoveries," but Doctor X has been gaining adherents over the years, and his fortunes are on the rise. Not because of his science, mind you, but mainly because the idea of genes regulating behavior in general is becoming more accepted. So he has some leverage.

Now he begins to research tissue samples of the seventeen carpenters; he has a new theory about how to analyze genes from those samples. This method is not known to 99% of human geneticists, but Doctor X has lots of equipment there in his lab, and seven people are necessary to run just several of the large machines at his disposal.

A period of silence ensues. Several years. At the end of this period, Doctor X wearily and in triumph emerges from his lab and tells the world, through the press, that he has once and for all isolated the suicide gene. In the cases of these seventeen carpenters, he has, moreover, discovered , in general at least, how the gene comes to be switched on.

Since he is backed by federal money, his pronouncements go unchallenged; it's clear that the scales have been tipped. More money is going to roll downhill towards Doctor X, and scientists want to be on the correct side of that incline. They're not stupid. They need research money, too.

Besides, more suicides are beginning to occur, and not just among carpenters. There is another group. Alaskan fishermen.

They're jumping off their boats in increasing numbers. Actually, all suicides in the US are up for the year.

Suicides in the U.S., Haiti, Africa, and Brazil are all up for the year. Doctor X publishes a paper indicating that these statistics are significant.

Already, people are beginning to ignore the first odd revelation that seventeen carpenters committed suicide. That is dropping out of the memory of most Americans. Hell, we seem to have an epidemic of sorts going on, one which embraces, or could come to embrace, the *globe*.

And now comes a sensational revelation. Artists in New York living below Houston Street are committing suicide too.

Doctor X appears on TV once every couple of months, assuring Americans that he is working on this devilish problem of trying to understand the complete mechanism by which the suicide gene is turned on. One thing, he stresses, is clear. There is a contagion of gene-activation. People are contacting other people, shaking hands, accidentally bumping shoulders, and the contact alone is somehow producing an interactive chemical effect which causes the suicide gene to activate. Therefore, on sheer probabilities, it is best to avoid crowds, and it is best to limit contacts with strangers.

Well, many people live by these principles anyway. So they were right all along. They just didn't know why.

Soon 80% of all grant monies being dished out by the feds to curb the new suicide epidemic are aimed at understanding the suicide gene better. Around the U.S., at universities, researchers are privately grumbling about Doctor X. How did he really prove that a single gene was responsible for suicide, and how did he prove that activation is created by personal contact involving a chemical triggering of some kind?

But the grumbling is private, because grant monies are at stake. Reputations can be broken by publicly taking Doctor X to task.

Rumors begin to ooze out of Doctor X's lab. X really has no way of verifying that his suicide gene controls suicide or has anything to do with that desperate act. X has been ranting of late against suggestions that exotic cofactors[1] , catalysts, might be involved in switching on the suicide gene.

"No cofactors!" he screams at least once a day. "All you need is the gene and simple chemical triggers. Suicide has nothing to do with anything else."

Several scientists actually come out into the open and say that the whole gene theory is sheer tripe, that suicide may not even be a single phenomenon to start with. That is, there may be vastly different reasons for ending one's own life, and the assumption that one suicide is exactly like another is absurd.

To which defenders of Doctor X scornfully reply: "We have an epidemic on our hands and these people are living in the dark ages with their multiple-cause theory. We have to do something right now about this revisitation of the black plague, and these gainsayers, professional critics, are trying to take us back into the past, back into ignorance. We have to move forward."

Of course, it is impossible to set up a controlled experiment to prove that Doctor X's gene causes suicide. If he's right, mechanical activation of the gene would cause immediate suicide. What experimental volunteer is going to stand still for that?

But many researchers point out that one aspect of the epidemic essentially proves Doctor X's theory is true:

Otherwise healthy New York bakers, who almost never, by actual count, commit suicide, have begun to kill themselves – and this has happened always after contact, on the lower East Side of NY, with high-risk artists and/or carpenters (whom they've contracted to do repairs in their shops).

What else does one need to prove, neatly and perfectly, in order to know finally that the suicide gene is alive and well and communicable?

But several researchers scratch a little below the surface and find that, of those bakers who apparently have come into contact with high-risk carpenters and artists, only 2% have committed suicide, and

---

[1] Cooperating elements (e.g. other germs, malnutrition, drugs) which enable a central germ or other factor to cause disease in a person.

some of those had terminal cancer. But this study is ignored by the researchers who are landing grants to study the suicide gene's mechanism.

In the next several years, there are more disturbing stories coming out of Doctor X's lab and adjoining labs. Doctor X is negotiating with several large pharmaceutical houses. He is thinking of leaving his position with the government and starting his own firm – the purpose of which will be to manufacture a drug which will directly interfere with the body chemicals that react when a high-risk person meets in public an unaware victim. What a boon this will be. By prophylactic use of this drug, a person will be able to walk the streets without fear. If he meets a high-risk person and the secret chemical contagion begins to occur – which would tragically switch on his own suicide gene – the new drug will stop all that.

Several more fringe researchers make accusations about Doctor X's plans to go into private drug-manufacture. This is essentially, they say, creating a conflict of interest: Dr. X is now committed to his (unproven) theory about the way the suicide gene is triggered, since he is planning to manufacture a drug to stop that triggering process.

In fact, a number of prominent scientists are now proposing other scenarios for how the suicide gene is switched on. Some think it happens by the transfer of a virus from person to person. The virus attacks the genome of certain nerve cells and triggers, accidentally, the suicide gene. Another story: the suicide gene turns on when the temperature of the brain rises beyond a certain point, and there could be many reasons for this heat-escalation, including ordinary fevers.

Wait a minute. We thought the map was already laid out. We thought it had definitely been proven that chemical reactions were set off in the victim when he contacted a high-risk person. If this part of the scenario is really up for grabs, then Doctor X's plans to go into private manufacture of a drug could *really* constitute an unconscionable bias – and since he is the number one government researcher on the subject of suicide . . . shouldn't he be disqualified and replaced?

Quietly, while Doctor X works in his lab trying to save us all, other developments are taking place which will dwarf what is occurring there. For the last several years, doctors and psychiatrists have been reporting all suicides as part of the growing epidemic. Previously, there had been some attempt to differentiate "ordinary suicides" committed for obvious down-to-earth human reasons from those triggered, most probably, by the gene after it was set off by contact with a high-risk person. But now, all that nicety has gone by the boards. ALL suicides are added to the rolls of the epidemic. Not only that, a pre-suicide state has been defined and diagnosed. No statistics are being kept, but it's estimated that 1.1 million Americans are in this pre-suicide state.

The symptoms? Restlessness, anxiety, depression. Whenever a doctor spots signs of these, he can make a presumptive pre-suicide diagnosis. Studies are beginning to show that, as time passes, more and more pre-S people are turning into actual suicide statistics.

Although no figures are released, beyond a specialized study of 3000 men from San Francisco, the word is, pre-S invariably leads to S. It's a death sentence. Of course, when a doctor makes the pre-S determination and so informs his patient, there is a strong hypnotic effect on the patient. Very strong.

Furthermore, patients with small pimples, with minor skin rashes, with headaches, with blurry vision from watching excessive amounts of TV, are flooding into doctors' offices, fearing the worst, that they are pre-S. A certain percentage leave the office with that diagnosis.

No one knows how long the incubation period is between pre-S and S.

But the capper comes when a friend and colleague of Doctor X makes this startling announcement in a televised press conference: murder is actually suicide.

Yes, an avalanche of studies undertaken over the last twenty years leave no doubt that a murderer is actually trying to kill himself. The act of killing is merely a mask for a biochemical event, the switching on of the suicide gene.

Suddenly, all of history takes on a new hue, a new weight. All those wars, those revolutions, those uprisings of the poor, those squashings of the peasants underheel, those poisonings of rivers by large thoughtless corporations – it's all a death wish, it's all suicide. It's all the same gene. It always was. It always will be.

If we thought we had an epidemic before, now the figures are monstrous. Every murder is now reported to the authorities as a suicide.

Now there is no turning back. No dissent is brooked. This death business is so horrible, so . . . *contagious* that we can't afford to debate strategies and underlying causes. We have to march forward in the groove established by the big-time researchers headed by Doctor X. The whole thrust of the program is now to give more money so we can progress faster. A cure must be found.

Villages, towns, cities, states are passing laws requiring the citizenry to submit to pre-S testing. Complaints that these "tests" are subjective and vague are squashed as counter-patriotic. Besides, we all know that murder and suicide are really undertaken by certain types of people, *and they are not like us.* They are genetically different, and who knows, maybe some day soon we'll be able to prove that they're genetically inferior.

In the meantime, detention centers are being set up so that those who show positive for the pre-S condition can be isolated. Speaking of isolation, in labs all over the country, chimps and gorillas and rhesus monkeys are being kept in sterile single isolation rooms where there is no sound, no motion, no germs. These primates have been operated on. Brain surgeries have been done, attempts to artifically switch on suicide genes, thus proving that Doctor X's thesis is true. Unfortunately, although one hundred plus primates have had the switching-on operation, none, after four-plus years, has killed himself.

There is some speculation, though, that the sterile isolation rooms may induce madness after enough years, which may in turn lead to suicide.

Insurance companies are funding research into the suicide-gene, and they are eagerly awaiting primate suicides. Their strategy is interesting: they hope to rule out, as uninsurable, all those people who are diagnosed as pre-S. After all, if a person is pre-S, while he is incubating his later suicide, he most probably will be prone to developing stress-related illnesses, which would ordinarily be covered by health plans. But if insurance companies can get away with refusing to insure pre-S types, they will go on in glorious days to develop complete genetic profiles of their applicants and thus be able to reject, forever, inferior specimens.

Needless to say, as time passes, the odd fate of the original seventeen suicidal carpenters, and others whose suicides really did seem to be unusual and a departure from pattern are ignored completely in the accumulating hysteria.

No one takes notice (and here, admittedly, I oversimplify) that the carpenters and the Alaskan fishermen and the artists are all using a new brand of shellack which contains a compound that makes airplane glue seem like room deodorizer. The destruction of brain cells upon inhalation of this shellack is nearly instantaneous and is quite extensive.

No one takes notice. Things are much too complicated now. With succeeding redefinitions of Suicide (even certain cancers are now being included under a category called Self-Created Terminal Conditions, in keeping with bland assurances of pop psychologists), one finds it very hard to go back in time and pick up vague threads.

In fact, pre-S seems to be the condition everyone is focusing on. There is no longer doubt that pre-S inevitably leads to S. The newspapers, TV, media pick up on the new assumption and incorporate it into their stories.

Since pre-S is so important now, little side-maladies are being defined that stick out from pre-S like spikes from an iron ball. First and foremost is pre-S schizophrenia (PSS). A psychiatrist at a leading Boston University publishes a list of early symptoms: sloppy hygiene; a sudden upsurge in attendance at church; crossing out names in one's telephone index; taking long walks alone; unbending paper clips; sudden anger; errors in paying taxes; a change in speaking intonation, according to neighbors; unreasoned fear of dentistry; discarding possessions; seeking to travel abroad for no apparent reason.

Several preachers who have not yet been found sleeping with prostitutes announce that these symptoms match one of the esoteric Bible prophecies. Yes, in the end-times, just before the Encounter on the Plain of Armageddon, sinners afflicted with plagues will begin to exhibit strange, baffling behaviors.

A new drug is introduced to treat those with pre-S. It is a cousin of ethyl chloride, which is already known to destroy brain cells every time it is inhaled. The new drug also attacks brain cells. It is thought that by permanently warping areas of the brain, the suicide gene might have no effect when it finally triggers. Of course, a state of considerable mental depreciation would already have taken place, from the drug therapy, but some life is better than none.

A spokesman for a large insurance company publicly disagrees. He is backing new detention legislation which will allow pre-S persons to ship out to any number of South Pacific atolls. In these colonies, one would be free from harassment by non pre-S types.

The U.S. intelligence community is busy making recommendations to the National Security Council. Since we are faced with a global epidemic, we should take advantage of the situation (before the other side does). The basic plan is simple. Foreign governments, particularly in lands bearing rich mineral reserves, should be wooed, with an eye toward their declaring national states of emergency, based on large numbers of pre-S citizens. U.S. medical representatives will assist. It will be made clear to these governments that no better way exists to cement national control than through medical channels. There are no political issues to promote, no ideologies to enunciate. All that's needed is the insistence of medical authorities that the Health Emergency dictates instituting curfews, postponing elections, and establishing detention centers for the afflicted.

Any connection between some of the afflicted and political dissidents is, of course, entirely coincidental.

Since casual personal contact with strangers can trigger the S-gene, no gathering of more than three persons in any public place will be tolerated.

Sex, a very personal form of contact, will be restricted to those couples registered as married.

Conceiving and giving birth will be subject to medical control, since Society must guard against pre-S mothers having pre-S babies.

"Tests are now being perfected" for detection of the S-gene in a state of near-triggering, but in the meantime, behavioral symptoms will be the guide. In this regard, a much larger list of early, intermediate, and late signs is being published. Some additions include: skin rashes; leathery patches on the face; speaking at excessive volume; losing objects; refusal to answer the telephone; a prolonged sober expression . . .

About this time, a confidential internal memorandum, written from an officer of a major pharmaceutical house to a member of the board, is leaked to the press. It causes a stir for a day or two, then sinks beneath the weight of new stories on pre-S.

From: HS
To: RY
Subject: Long Term Planning; What Sort of Research Grant Shall We Fund in the Future?

The ideal disease, from a financial point of view, RY, would be one in which the entire catalog of human symptoms were interlocked. In other words, you could start from a sore throat, and know that all sore throats were nothing more than ominous pre-conditions for the emergence of heavier symptoms, like fever, like lowered T-cells counts. These, in turn, would be locked on to another heavier branch of the disease-tree, which involved malaise, melancholy, despondence.

And each branch of symptoms would involve tests to ascertain the exactness of the patient's medical position.

On each branch, there would exist various drugs, various remedies. Each drug would have toxic side-effects in various degrees, and would invoke its own symptoms, which would show up later in more serious well-defined elements of the disease, further down toward the trunk of the tree.

Ultimately, once you arrived on the trunk you would have a congealing of psychological and physical symptoms requiring surgical removal of organs, including, at last, the brain, which would be used for further research on the one Disease.

Each new definitional phase of the Disease would of course involve the office-visit for the diagnosis, and that diagnosis would give the patient a jolt of depression. It would also, by dint of education, give him knowledge of the whole tree, bit by bit. He would *know* that his current symptoms were indicative of worse things to come. A sore throat would never be a sore throat. It would be a prelude to probable disaster and would function, to a degree, as a self-fulfilling prophecy.

As I say, business-wise, this is the ideal Disease. The interlocking of all human symptoms requiring more invasive intervention and, thus, compounding side-effects. The opposite extreme would be a sniffle that was regarded merely as a sniffle. . .

CHAPTER TWENTY-TWO

AIDS MEDIA ON THE POLITICAL RIGHT

Here are a few examples of a different sort of news coverage and media play on AIDS.

Under the banner headline *AIDS?* on the cover of the newspaper for the Moral Majority, *Liberty Report* (May 1987), the following short text is printed over the space of half the page: "And in the same way also the men abandoned the natural function of the woman and burned in their desire towards one another, men with men committing indecent acts and receiving in their own persons the due penalty of their error. Romans 1:27 New American Standard."

In an undated release titled, "FROM ME TO YOU by Jimmy Swaggart/ IS AIDS A JUDGMENT FROM GOD?", Swaggart writes, "Every baby that contracts AIDS through a blood transfusion, etc. can thank the homosexual community for his death. Likewise, every individual who receives contaminated blood while undergoing surgery can thank the homosexual community for his death."

Swaggart's group mails out an issue of *The Evangelist* (December, 1987) as well. Written by Don Boys, preacher, a former member of the Indiana House of Representatives, its text is similar to other work from the religious right:

1) "God warned mankind about AIDS in Numbers 32:23 when He said, '*Be sure your sin will find you out.*'"

2) "In every formal debate and every television talk show dealing with sodomy that I have been involved with, I have always heard the old lie about the great contributions creative homosexuals have made to society. But they never tell the whole truth and nothing but the truth. They only shine the spotlight on a few well-known perverts that made a name for themselves, and those are debatable."

3) "The sodomite doesn't tell you that it is not the upper and middle classes of people who are sodomites, but the lower classes of people. The prisons are full of them. Homosexual rape is the norm for most prisons. Officials look the other way."

4) "Sodomites are the most vicious people in the world. Many of the mass murders have been committed by sodomites . . . Out of 518 deaths in the past 17 years, sodomites killed 350 of them — 68 percent (and remember that homosexuals make up only about 4 percent of the population)."

5) "As a member of the Indiana House of Representatives, I introduced a bill to make sodomy illegal again . . . They acted as if I wanted to hang them from the maples on the statehouse lawn, but all I wanted to do was put them in jail from 7 to 21 years (as we had been doing in Indiana for 75 years)."

6) "Dr. Robert Benjamin is reported in *Newsweek* (September 13,1985, issue) as saying, 'To completely control AIDS you would have to quarantine people for life.' Well, get to it if that is necessary."

Bible historian James McKeever, who appears on the cover of one of his books with Pat Robertson, has penned *The AIDS Plague* (Omega Publications, 1986). The introduction was written by Dr. Ralph Byron, former chief of surgery at the City of Hope Hospital. Byron writes, "In the final analysis, I believe the only adequate solution for AIDS is a vital faith in the resurrected Christ!"

McKeever takes a softer tone than, say, Jimmy Swaggart. However, by page 17 he is making this suggestion: "A military base...goes to 'Condition Red' when harm is imminent. There is no panic at a Red Alert, but there is serious concern and acute alertness.

"It is time to declare a state of national health emergency concerning AIDS."

McKeever suggests HIV testing for everyone in America. He thinks people might be tagged in three categories, stage 0, 1 and 2. At 0 (antibody-negative) you would be issued a green card. At 1 (antibody-positive), you would be issued a yellow card. If you were both antibody-positive and had symptoms, stage 2, you would get a red card. He also discusses giving "infected" students their lessons at home by video (". . . AIDS may force us to move to a more isolated type of education technology.")

Finally, in Appendix B to the book, McKeever gets rolling and offers four steps to being healed from one of God's plagues. A person must humble himself, really pray, seek God's face, and turn from wicked ways. As AIDS turns into an opportunity to enforce morality, McKeever makes his ultimate pitch in a section headed, "PROTECTION DEPENDENT UPON OBEDIENCE." He defines a state of voluntary slavery (bondslavery) and says that a bondslave is a "volunteer permanent slave."

"Here we see," McKeever writes, "that God seals His bond-slaves...on their foreheads. Later we find out why: He seals them for their protection against the plagues coming upon the earth." Message: Become a slave to God and He will save you from AIDS.

It's easy to believe that the influence of hawkish right-wing Christianity is on the wane, its cartoonish aspects shunted to one side of the American stage. But the failure to understand this bizarre world-view, this closed system of faith and thought, leaves us all prone to disaster.

Those who make a living out of analyzing and reporting on American society don't want to get too close to the religious right -- they are afraid their colleagues will somehow make them guilty by association, particularly if they give the movement its due: It is the most important political force in America in the last twenty-five years. It will continue to have an important role in the next administration.

Here is a particularly interesting bit of wisdom from Jerry Falwell, who has hosted events for his friend George Bush, and told crowds that Bush is the man for the White House in 1988:

Falwell: "You'll be riding along in an automobile. You'll be the driver perhaps. You're a Christian. There'll be several people in the automobile with you, maybe someone who is not a Christian. When the trumpet sounds, you and other born-again believers in that automobile will be instantly caught away -- you will disappear, leaving behind only your clothes and physical things that cannot inherit eternal life. The unsaved person or persons in the automobile will suddenly be startled to find that the car is moving along without a driver, and the car suddenly somewhere crashes . . . Other cars on the highways driven by believers will suddenly be out of control and stark pandemonium will occur on . . . every highway in the world where Christians are caught away (taken to heaven) from the driver's wheel."

This sort of astonishing occurrence, according to Falwell and other American luminaries of the religious right, e.g., Pat Robertson[1] and Jimmy Swaggart and Billy Graham, marks a period called the Rapture, during which born-again Christians will be swept away into heaven, body and soul, by Jesus.

What then follows on Earth is a terrible period called the Tribulation, marked by land war, nuclear exchanges between the U.S. and the USSR, disease, pain and general all-around suffering. This is what you get if you're not born-again, and it may explain the strange glint in these preachers' eyes on Sunday morning TV. They believe they know something we don't.

They know that Armageddon is on the horizon, because the Bible tells them so -- if it's read selectively, of course. And one of the most obvious signs of the end of history is plagues. AIDS.

A 1985 Nielsen survey showed that 61 million Americans regularly listen to preachers who tell them nuclear war is a fact in our generation.

Pat Robertson, the broadcaster and candidate for President in 1988, spoke to 16 million families every day on television, or 20% of Americans who own TVs. His 700 Club brings in $200 million a year, reaching a group that is larger than the readership of the *New York Times, LA Times, Washington Post, Time* and *Newsweek* combined.

Jimmy Swaggart, White House visitor and TV preacher, spoke to 4.5 million households daily, Jerry Falwell talks to 5.6 million households. Both have been regular White House guests.

The vast majority of 80,000 religious broadcasters who speak to the nation every day on radio and TV believe in nuclear Armaged-

---

[1] Robertson believes Christians must suffer the end of the world down here, after which the Kingdom of God will be established.

don. The technical term is *dispensationalism*. As in, God dispensing justice. AIDS, of course, being one of God's very important dispensations.

There are 10,000 Americans in Bible colleges today. Upon graduating they will move to proselytizing, teaching, starting their own Bible colleges.

People with end-times scenarios are very conscious of AIDS and view it in that symbolic light. For these types, an epidemic is a perfect hook. They can come in behind it with much business about purity and detainment of the impure.

These harder elements of the religious right definitely accept nuclear war and other signs of the end-times such as AIDS. They mean God's final prophecies are coming to pass. And of course, in the later fullness of time, when Jesus does return to Earth to set up his kingdom of a thousand years of peace, he'll bring with him all those born-agains he snatched out of their cars on the freeway. They'll be executives and white collar workers in the new paradise.

There are, of course, big dollars to be made from television preaching, and, yes, there is great power to wield over flocks of the eager, and yes, there is the sweet idea of revenge against the sinners -- revenge in knowing that God will burn them in oil forever, and soon. But to understand these people of the religious right, you have to understand the ecstasy of the "visionary."

The question is, why would a preacher making $100 million a year seriously believe in and welcome the end of the world? He'd be too busy enjoying his money to want it all to end. This is the point at which many critics of these preachers just call it all a shuck and dismiss the movement.

But here is a clue. Ramrodded by a desire to get revenge on the sinners of our times, dispensationalists believe that when they go, when they are taken up into the sky by Jesus at the End, before the bombs go off down here on Earth, they will keep their bodies with them; this isn't just an ethereal ascension. There is form too. The manicured nails, the coiffed hair, the straightened teeth. This is survival of a distinctly new kind, unknown to science or even to mystical religions of the past.

And Christian Heaven, as anyone can see from a cursory tour of cathedrals, is, as Alan Watts once said, "a very extravagant place. God doesn't *need* all those servants around Him, He's omnipotent, but he likes the flitting cherubs and the angels and the singing and the baroque curlicues. The whole kingdom in the clouds."

The fact is, Falwell and others believe they will travel to Heaven first class, and if that doesn't beat it all, what will?

The trip with Jesus will lead them back here to rule in his kingdom for a thousand years. Do you think Jerry Falwell or Ronald Reagan see themselves as dishwashers in the new paradise? Do you think they see themselves minus perks in the New World? No, they belive they won't lose a thing.

You *can* take it with you.

And you can live in a Disney heaven on earth, cleared of all the riff-raff.

These people see religion as essentially a military campaign waged by the greatest general of all time, Jesus Christ, pronouncements about laying down the sword and turning the other cheek notwithstanding. He will lead his troops to victory over Satan in the greatest Superbowl ever played. It is no wonder that the military mind is fascinated by the evangelical position. No wonder that the Pentagon and the intelligence services are replete with born-agains.

And with people like George Bush (born-again) and Pat Robertson waiting in the wings, the religious beat will go on.

Caressing the idea that God is going to wage nuclear war, bring down fire and brimstone among us mortals, is like the ultimate game of chicken, the ultimate fraternity hazing stunt among men of religious right. They are awed by those with the most apparent disregard of life and limb, the Olivers of Norths. Men with guns and God behind them are the biggest kick in the world to these men of the cloth -- and Armageddon itself is the biggest game of war.

Somewhere in their souls, Falwell, Reagan, Robertson are in love with nuclear clouds ballooning and expanding out over populations. This is *power*.

We said these preachers were stupid. They were sick, they were conning the socks off poor saps in Virginia and Mississippi.

Meanwhile they're having lunch at the White House. Falwell is being briefed by the National Security Council on our nuclear strategies vis-a-vis the Russians, and Hal Lindsey, modern guru of Armegeddon, author of *The Late Great Planed Earth*, is addressing Pentagon generals on the waging of nuclear war. These things have happened.

Considerable propaganda about AIDS has gone out among congregations and TV audiences of the religious right. As we are now in the year of a Presidential campaign, there is the question of how to approach the AIDS issue and squeeze the most political mileage out of it for a Geroge Bush.

The note at the moment is one of caution. But that is only a strategic matter. Given possible future escalation of public sentiment against so-called high risk groups, given what might become a correct moment in a wave of public hysteria about AIDS, the religious right would move more boldly in the public arena -- and their potential should not be tossed off. They have both money and organization in considerable amounts, and through political action committees and fund raising organizations, they have completely emerged out of the bumpkin-phase in Washington politics.

In the fall of 1987, the *Bay Area Reporter*, a San Francisco paper, uncovered a confidential memorandum which may have been passed within an outfit called Charlton Research. Charlton is a PR firm that has done work for the Republican Party. The *Reporter* stated that Chuck Rund, who was a deputy manager of Ronald Reagan's 1984 campaign, wrote the memo. Rund denies this. He says a former aide, unhappy with his job, wrote and leaked it to the *Reporter*. The February 1988 *Harper's* reprinted the memo. It's instructive to read, because it assumes that strategy and winning are the only real considerations in how hard to press the AIDS issue:

September 17, 1987

187

AIDS INC.

TO: HD
FROM: CR
RE: AIDS Issue

The AIDS issue could easily be a paramount one in 1988. It is important that it be used effectively and wisely. It is an explosive issue that could easily backfire if (handled) in a heavy or blatant way.

Nationally, SRC (Senate Republican Committee), the Bush campaign, the Washington governor campaign, and the Robertson campaign are exploring ways to harness public reation to the AIDS issue. It will be used in major races in both Texas and Florida.

In California it is a mixed bag. Some Republicans, Maddy (a Republican state senator), Quackenbush (an aide to Republican governor George Deukmejian), refuse to try and exploit it, but many are more than willing. If we do, we *must* be discreet. An example of how not to approach it is Congressman Dannemeyer (R., Calif.). At the meeting two weeks ago, he was terrifying -- practically foaming at the mouth anytime anyone made even a sympathetic reference to people with AIDS. Someone like Dannemeyer is a live grenade on this issue and far too emotional to do any good; indeed I fear that he would scare a lot of people.[2]   (Republican state senator) Doolittle's approach is far better: sound reasonable, play the emotion, and above all make it appear is if the party is responding to a public ground swell rather than inciting one. We must avoid being labeled as extremists; the recent fate of the La Rouche and the Briggs initiatives (Republican state senator John Briggs introduced a bill in the state legislature to prohibit gays from teaching in public schools) prove that an outright attack will be rejected by the voters.

This is the plan for the (Democratic state senator) Garamandi campaign. We shall make contact with various pro-life, family organizations and have them launch campaigns. In Garamandi's district,

---

[2] Dannemeyer states he did not attend the meeting in question, he did not foam at the mouth, and the memo is a fictitious document.

the Century Assembly of God Church seems a likely ally. They are hardworking, politically ignorant, but as zealous as Dannemeyer. Attacking Garamandi as Pro-Abortion, Pro-Gay and therefore Pro-AIDS might prove to be easy.

Not only could the AIDS issue help us to gain ground in '88, but it might help us hang on (in places) where some of our people are in trouble (Dornan [R., Calif.]). *Again, the Republican party must never seem to be inciting a reaction, only responding to it.* If we are low-key, sound logical, and stress the importance of "protecting" families from the disease, then we could find ourselves in excellent shape in '88.

In February of 1988, I interviewed the pastor of a church south of Los Angeles on the subject of AIDS. The pastor had, for some time, been telling his flock that AIDS was "a disease and a plague sent from God to signal that we were in the end-times, that sinners were going to suffer for their crimes."

During the interview, which took several turns that the pastor didn't like, he said he was only going to continue talking off the record. Here is an excerpt from our conversation:

Q: What is AIDS?

A: It is a punishment for acts done against the idea of the family and religion.

Q: And how is that plague introduced?

A: You mean, on the physical plane?

Q: Yes.

A: Through the AIDS virus.

Q: God sent it through the green monkey in Africa?

A: Maybe. That's what they say.

Q: The scientists.

A: Yes.

Q: They say there are several of these AIDS viruses now.

A: Well, God would send several plagues, but it's all AIDS.

Q: Do you know there are people who have been to a number of bisexual swing clubs in New York and other cities, and have reported all kinds of sex going on between men and men, and men and women? Why didn't the HIV virus spread out into the hetero community at that point and cause AIDS in a big way?

A: Why should it?

Q: Because it's a virus. That's what viruses do, don't they?

A: I can't answer that.

Q: Did God make contagious HIV that only affected male gays and IV drug users in America, and then affected black African heterosexuals in Africa?

A: You mean a virus that stopped at the boundaries of certain groups.

Q: Why would a virus do that ?

A: My understanding is that viruses don't do that.

Q: That's correct.

A: I've always thought the Soviets might have had some part in this.

Q: You mean, they are making an attempt to destroy America with AIDS?

A: Yes.

Q: And God is working through the Russians.

A: (laughs) I don't think God works through them.

Q: But you said that God had invented the AIDS virus. I thought just now you meant that God gave the Soviets the idea of the HIV virus, and showed them how to make it in one of their labs. And the the Soviets spread it to America.

A: No. The Soviets would do that on their own.

Q: The Soviets would be trying to destroy America with AIDS. Since AIDS, you say, affects only the sinners in America, then the Soviets would have invented a virus to lay waste to sinners in America.

A: No.

Q: That would make America stronger, by getting rid of all the sinners.

A: You see, AIDS is a plague. This is where you have to start, in order to understand it. A plague from God.

Q: So God is also punishing the Haitians and Africans in Central Africa, and people in Brazil.

A: These people have been lax for a long time, in a way.

Q: In what way.

A: They don't become technologically advanced, like the rest of the world.

Q: And this is a sin.

A: It creates a kind of drag on the rest of society. We then have to help these people with money and food and machines.

Q: And because of this drag, God sent them a plague.

A: They don't believe in Jesus, either, despite the many efforts of missionaries.

Q: The ones that do would be spared.

A: If they believe in their hearts.

Q: Most sinners in America are men?

A: Why should that be?

Q: Because, of all reported AIDS cases, 91% are men.

A: That could be a mistake.

Q: In statistics?

A: Yes.

Q: Are you familiar with the approved treatment for AIDS, AZT?

A: Yes, it's a drug that's been around for one or two years now.

Q: Some people who take it then need blood transfusions. AZT also can have adverse effects on bone marrow.

A: Well, this could be a further punishment.

Q: You mean God working through the medical establishment?

A: Not exactly. The scientists are correct in their assessments of the situation, as far as they are able to comprehend it.

Q: Would God, for example, punish homosexuals in New York but not in Des Moines or other cities where AIDS hasn't developed to any great extent?

A: In the large cities, the drug-using and sexual activities are more pronounced.

Q: Why haven't there been many cases of AIDS in China, the Soviet Union, and other Communist countries?

A: Because they keep their borders closed to outsiders.

Q: God wouldn't cross borders? If Communism is closely linked to atheism, why hasn't God visited AIDS in a big way on those countries? Is there a ranking of sin, according to which is worst?

A: There may be. There is. Sometimes we humans have trouble understanding it.

Q: Well, for instance, would male homosexuality be worse than lesbianism?

A: It's hard to choose, in that case.

Q: Because cases of reported AIDS among lesbians are nearly non-existent.

A: That may have something to do with the virus itself.

Q: In what way?

A: It may be suited to men.

Q: You know this?

A: No, I'm just suggesting that...You see, when a person has family values, real values, all these questions become clear, in so far as society is concerned.

Q: How does that happen?

A: Well, when you have a family to protect, you see the dangers. You may not understand the little pieces of this plague, but you see how it generally affects people trying to maintain a clean family.

Q: In this year's Presidential race, would you say that voters concerned with these family values would recognize the right candidates?

A: You mean, the candidate that was against the spread of AIDS into families? Yes. That would be obvious.

Q: And the right candidate would be Bush?

A: I don't tell my congregation how to vote.

Q: Would you be in favor of quarantining those people who test positive for the HIV virus?

A: It may come to that, if this thing gets more serious.

Q: And you would support that.

CHAPTER TWENTY-TWO

A: As a public health measure, if we had to do it, yes.

Q: But you believe that AIDS only affects those who are sinners. It isn't just a random thing?

A: Oh no. A plague truly is a sign. It tells you that, in this case, sinners are afflicted, and the end of history is over the horizon. But the end of history isn't necessarily a bad thing.

Q: But the sinners have to be punished.

A: Yes, otherwise there wouldn't be Heaven on Earth later on.

Q: As minister to your congregation, would you urge them all to get tested for HIV?

A: Only if they were homosexual or IV drug users, and I don't think we have any of those.

Q: In other words, those are the sins which God would punish by sending down HIV.

A: Those are the people who can spread HIV.

Q: But nobody else can.

A: That's what we're told.

Q: But in a religious sense, is this a plague just to punish homosexuality and needle-drugs?

A: That would be much too limited, don't you think?

Q: Well, if there are other sins that God could punish with HIV, what would they be? Adultery? Sleeping with prostitutes? Watching pornographic films?

A: Sleeping with prostitutes, yes.

Q: So, if any of your congregation have done that, on business trips or the like, then they should be tested too.

A: If we have any of those.

Q: And these preachers we hear about who have been sleeping with women they weren't married to, should they be tested?

A: Why not?

Q: If they tested positive, should they be put in detention? Quarantine?

A: Well, I would leave that to God. I wouldn't judge.

Q: So HIV is basically a plague for the sin of illicit sex. Except for the case of IV drugs.

A: It seems that way.

Q: Maybe the reason there aren't a lot of AIDS cases in the Soviet Union has to do with less fooling around. Sexually.

A: I wouldn't know. But their basic sin is rejecting God and Jesus Christ. That would be more a spiritual thing. So they may be afflicted in other ways.

Q: Maybe mental ways. Some dementia, perhaps.

A: Yes. Possibly.

Q: One or two scientists have come out and said that the HIV virus doesn't infect enough cells to cause harm to the body.

A: I hadn't heard that. Maybe, if that's true, the virus has another way of working in the body.

Q: What would that be?

A: I wouldn't know. But again, this is God, so to speak, so He would have a way of making the thing behave according to His laws.

Q: The thing? The virus?

A: That's right.

Q: Let's suppose that no one has proved AIDS is a single thing, a single global epidemic. Could you accept that?

A: You see, where we are getting off the track here, I'm speaking with knowledge of the Bible, and you aren't. The Bible makes it clear that we are in the end-times. That's to me the power of certain passages in the Bible. No one can absolutely guarantee that we are the last generation, but I see it and others see it in these Biblical prophecies and analogies. Therefore, we know that plagues are here and they are part of that picture. So regardless of what people say, the plague is here. It's the right time.

Q: The science, then, doesn't make much difference.

A: Whether one scientist says this and another says that is just debate and argument. We can see that AIDS is a plague, those of us who study the Bible.

194

CHAPTER TWENTY-THREE

MANDATORY TESTING/DETAINMENT

A complete accounting of all state laws which pertain to AIDS, through 1987, would require a formidable research effort. The Intergovernmental Health Policy Project at George Washington University has summarized AIDS laws from 1987 state legislative sessions. To my knowledge, they are the only group which has an overview.

From their study, one can see, for example, that 13 states have some form of mandatory testing (HIV) for specialized groups: food handlers, hospital patients, couples about to be married, newborn children, prisoners, and prostitutes.

Nine states allow for some form of isolation/quarantine.

Nine states require some form of reporting/surveillance for those "infected" with HIV.

It is clear that, as of yet, no state is pushing for massive quarantine. Certain commissioners of health, however, have the flexibility to take actions they deem necessary for public health. That may involve co-approval by boards of health, or governors, or legislatures. In some cases, commissioners have unequivocal power to act alone.

All states have completely bought the assumption that AIDS is a classical sexually transmitted disease, and that the HIV test is a good indicator of present infection by the causative agent of the disease.

If you could freeze time and read AIDS laws, you would conclude that most states are being cautious on matters of detention for "HIV carriers."

But time is not frozen. Events can lead to a defusing of hysteria about AIDS or an escalation. In the latter case, these laws will be gradually pressed into service. The last three years tell you this has already been happening to a degree.

AIDS INC.

Here is an example, from the Intergovernmental Health Policy Project 1987 summary, of a few current state laws:

1) Alabama HB 338 – "Provides for commitment proceedings for those infected with notifiable diseases or designated STDs (e.g., AIDS) who refuse testing and treatment and for those who, by their conduct, put others at risk of infection . . . Those responsible for reporting known or *suspected* cases include physicians, dentists . . . school principals and day care center directors." (emphasis added)

Not reporting is subject to a $100-500 fine.

It is interesting that principals and day care directors are invested with medical acumen by law; and can a person be detained for refusing, say AZT?

In North Dakota, SB 2117 "expands the powers and duties of the State Health Officer to include issuing orders relating to disease control measures necessary to prevent the spread of communicable diseases (e.g., AIDS). Disease control measures may include special immunization activities and decontamination measures . . . cancelling public events or closing places of business (with District Court approval.)"

Oregon HB2067 "provides that, whenever a local public health administrator reasonably believes a person may have a communicable disease (e.g., AIDS) . . . the person may be ordered to be examined. The order is to include a statement that the person may refuse to submit to an examination, in which case a public health measure may be imposed, including isolation, quarantine or other preventive health measure (providing certain guidelines and due process provisions are followed) . . ."

A final note for now: the late Dr. Robert Mendelsohn's *The People's Doctor*, a consumer newsletter (vol. 12, no. 2), reports that "the world's first AIDS colony (a 16th-century manor) is being established on the island of Adelso, near Stockholm, Sweden...there men and women (AIDS patients) will be confined in an escape-proof compound behind three-meter thick walls patrolled by armed

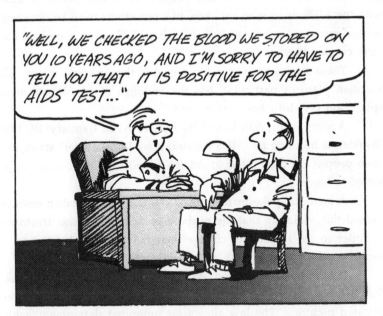

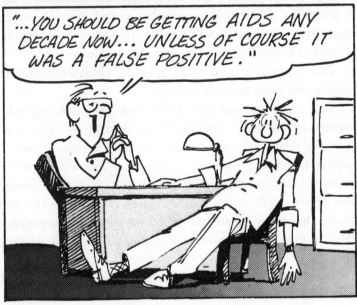

guards...Since 1985, Swedish law has stipulated that people infected with the AIDS virus who are likely to infect others must be detained." Several reports also indicate that, in Cuba, AIDS patients are held on a farm outside Havana.

These stories have been low-keyed in the American press. The Swedish plan, in particular, has the makings of an obvious news splash; yet very little has been printed.

A story in the Salt Lake City *Deseret News* (January 19, 1988, "Sweden is building an 'AIDS Alcatraz'," by Ron Laytner) states that, once people are committed to Adelso Island, they will never be allowed to leave.

A medical spokesman at the Washington DC Swedish embassy denied this, claiming that the purpose of detainment was treatment, in order to get inmates to change their irresponsible behavior. At most, he said, a stay on the island would last two months.

However, George Sved, coordinator for the Stockholm-based Swedish Federation for Sexual Equality, painted a slightly more complicated picture: "The law allows for unlimited detainment, which ends when the doctor is convinced his patient will follow sound medical advice about not spreading HIV. However, no real treatment is planned to achieve this end during the detention period."

This suggests a door could open for behavior modification techniques and other aversive "therapy."

This year's International AIDS Conference is being held in Stockholm, in June. The Social Democratic Party, Sved said, "is planning to use their model for dealing with HIV-positive people as a showpiece for visiting nations . . . There are extreme political elements in the country, although at present they don't have strong influence on the AIDS issue. The EAP party, connected with Lyndon LaRouche, has a few agents here proposing permanent separation of so-called healthy people from the infected. An example is Doctor Lita Tibling."

The *Deseret News* article contained several quotes from Tibling: "I would put all who test HIV positive on the island in small communities for life so they can't spread the infection. As far as their families visiting: I would put them all on the island too. They are probably already infected . . . as the AIDS plague worsens, the world's attitude will harden in a year or two.

"We must have national testing. Polls show that 70% of the Swedish people want compulsory testing . . . I believe Sweden will be the first country with compulsory testing – probably this year."

An anonymous source at the U.S. federal level states that the Adelso Island detainment scheme is part of a larger plan which is being viewed with interest by Western nations. In phase one, all Swedes would be tested for HIV, given health cards indicating their status. HIV positive people who are IV drug users, prostitutes, or people who lead promiscuous lifestyles (homosexual or heterosexual) would be detained. If it was then determined that a person would not change his behavior, he would be sent to Adelso Island.

Phase one might also entail restrictions on foreigners coming into Sweden.

Phase two, according to this source, would be much more extreme. It would involve detention colonies for all HIV-positive people and their families, the possible closure of national borders and even government approval before having a baby.

Whether phase two is just one of those theoretical bureaucratic contingency plans or a real program is hard to determine.

Personally, talking with people in the US about the detainment facility in Sweden leads me to believe that there is some support for this kind of idea. Hypnotized completely by HIV, there are people who, though not willing to actively support detention, will express approval when they hear someone else is trying it.

CHAPTER TWENTY-FOUR

ACTIVIST STRATEGIES

Convincing federal health agencies to act responsibly flies in the face of tradition established at those agencies which goes back a long way.

Take cancer.

One of its basic myths is that it, too, like AIDS, is a unity. The special viral cancer project in the 1970s tried to unify cancer even further by finding a germ that did it all. That project acquired knowledge but ultimately failed. Demanding a single cure for cancer did not do the trick, and in a similar though not identical sense, demanding a single cure for AIDS will not work because *health*, consistently good immune-response, is much more than the relief medical drugs bring from acute symptoms.

Medicine has been built to respond to acute crisis in the body. Under that aegis, it has extended its writ into the territory of "health maintenance," for which it really has no program.

When researchers assure people that AIDS is invariably fatal and that it is caused in toto by the HIV virus, they are instructing us on a philosophy of medicine. This kind of thinking is what people are trying to bloat with more research money. It's not going to work.

Activists seeking a solution to AIDS may end up doing a lot more than forcing the medical research establishment to accelerate research. They may force a revolution in the idea of what health care is. That is one of the things medical bureaucrats are nervous about.

A case in point is the intervention of the Massachusetts Attorney General in the affairs of Ann Wigmore. A Boston resident, Wigmore has for years headed up the local Hippocrates Health Institute. Attorney General Shannon has enjoined her from claiming she can cure AIDS with a two-week course of "energy soup," which is made out of sprouts.

Wigmore denies having said she could cure AIDS.

Attorney General Shannon is also trying to stop Wigmore from selling a booklet written by her "in which she contends she can strengthen and rebuild a patient's immune system," writes the *Boston Globe* (Jan.20, 1988).

The Massachusetts injunction is absurd. In a perfect world, perhaps AMA/NIH/CDC powers-that-be might be able to display marvelously clean hands and lucid minds and go on to criticize an outsider's poor health advice, but in this world, in 1988, the energy soup is a hell of a lot less harmful than many pharmaceuticals. Apparently though, the US Constitution contains a little known clause which empowers medical bureaucrats, through existing law enforcement agencies, to define at will the concept *cure* by banning literature on the subject.[1]

In various states, AIDS quackery commissions are being formed by Justice Departments in concert with local medical associations. Physicians who treat AIDS patients are being trained to adhere to the party line, which is that the only acceptable treatment for AIDS is AZT.

This is, of course, preposterous, in light of the fact that medicine has no tradition of being able to treat the immune system on a long-term basis, to bring it back to good condition. On this ground of no knowledge, Medicine has little to offer, little reason to set itself up as an authority. (As if reason mattered.)

At every level of media, there is silence on these elements of the current AIDS scene. Again, this is because it's assumed Medicine is right. Investigating this arena is a no-priority item for newspapers.

I believe the following strategies, some of which are now in place among activist groups, would help reduce hysteria and put things in perspective:

1) Bring a case to court which will test HIV as the cause of AIDS; subpoena the right scientists and start challenging the issue.

---

[1] Now, as of April, 1988, Wigmore has been told she is free to sell her book.

2) Campaign against mandatory HIV testing wherever it is threatened, and against detainment based on HIV tests. Challenge and refute the scientific credibility of the test. (See Chapter 31.)

3) Educate Congress on the expansion of the AIDS empire, how the concept of immune suppression is being linked worldwide, pinned to a single virus, and milked for pharmaceutical money.

4) Challenge the idea that AIDS is invariably fatal, or that a positive HIV test necessarily leads to illness.

5) Demand the firing of the team that lost the war on cancer at NIH, starting with Robert Gallo, and open up the research on AIDS to other causative scenarios.

6) Pressure university biologists to speak out against the monolithic grip on AIDS research at the top of the ladder, and the climate of fear that pervades the scene, wherein scientists are reluctant to disagree with top AIDS research-groups because their grant monies might dry up.

7) Encourage the formation of new private foundations to research methods of reducing immune suppression.

8) Demand jail terms for pharmaceutical executives who allow dangerous, immunosuppressive drugs and pesticides to be sold in the Third World.

9) Seeing that AIDS has been defined as most if not all human immunosuppression, lobby for a sweeping international investigation of medical, biowarfare, and animal research centers. Not only should all biowarfare research be terminated, internationally, as a lunatic preoccupation, but scientists working in the mystical sanctuaries of animal and medical labs must prepare themselves for a lengthy period of scrutiny, in which their methods, safety procedures, and results will be thrown open to public view. *Demand an assessment of NIH results in the last twenty years of its medical research.*

If such a list of actions seems excessively weighty, I can only defend it by saying that the uninspected history of immunosuppression is also weighty.

If such a list of actions, on the other hand, seems impossible to carry out, because no truly objective panel backed up law enforcement personnel can be gathered, then that is just a signal that things are as bad as some imagine.

If supporting such actions ever appealed to the media, in more adventuresome days, now our papers, our television networks, even most of our magazines are wedded to the idea that a news story does not even exist unless an official agency/body/organization announces it. In short, the planet itself could be splitting in half, and unless a committee of scientists told a paper, and unless a government agency confirmed it, a news editor would tell his reporter on the scene that the elephant who holds up the world is only suffering temporary back-spasms.

But if a Scopes trial on HIV could be brought into court, if the scientists could be subpoenaed, if the lawyers were million-dollar babies, reporters would show up and the story would be covered.

Some gay activists feel that debunking HIV as the cause of AIDS will set back the clock, and bring more intense blame for AIDS on the "gay lifestyle." That is an issue that can be handled and overcome. What is much harder to overcome is the perpetuation of the idea of a viral plague, one that is sweeping the world and carrying populations in its path. The *longer* AIDS is perpetuated in people's minds, and made more frightening, the more blame is going to accrue to so-called high risk groups. That is the real problem, and the media are cooperating entirely with this HIV plague-image of AIDS.

Were AIDS broken into various types and instances of immunosuppression, were the real factors, many of which I've described, identified for the public, the fear would recede.

As long as media blithely believe they are getting the straight dope from federal health agencies, they will keep building this absurd myth. They will keep bumbling along, believing they are documenting the earnest struggle of a hardy band of researchers against a plague caused by HIV. This is the way they've documented every campaign against a major disease. Why change now? Just do another re-run.

In the midst of this image-making, the simple facts get buried.

They are:

Every year or two, the bureaucratic gods of the CDC invent a new shotgun. The shotgun has wider barrels and more firepower, and what the gun spews out is a new definition of AIDS.

In the process, of course, pellets do land on people who have unusual disease problems, but the overall effect is to generate confusion and fear. By an interesting circumstance, larger disease-definitions equal larger drug profits.

Such flim-flam allows a company like Burroughs-Wellcome to sink $80 million into researching AZT, a drug that adversely affects bone marrow and causes serious anemia. The drug is marketed for $8,000-10,000 per year, per patient, and pretty soon doctors are handing it out like rosewater.

Back in 1980, when the first five AIDS patients-to-be showed up at Los Angeles hospitals, they were misdiagnosed. They did have pneumocystis carinii pneumonia and several other infections. But as any doctor should have been able to tell, pneumocystis can occur when there is immune suppression *for virtually any reason*. That is the history of the disease. Unexplainably stunned that these Los Angeles patients were immunocompromised, doctors made noises about a new syndrome, and pretty soon (in about ten seconds, I believe it was) everybody forgot that the name of the restaurant these ill men had eaten at was Inhalant Nitrites and Other Chemicals. The search for a virus was on.

Soon, a fairy tale arose about Africa and its green monkeys: The virus had come from them. Since green monkey kidneys had been used for years in making vaccines, since the monkeys themselves had been stretched, bent, poked, sliced, isolated and experimented on in laboratories all over the world, naturally AIDS *couldn't* have come from vaccines or labs – only from the African jungle.

Based on green monkey thinking, Africa was taken into the AIDS family, and soon the whole Third World was absorbed. The newly defined symptoms were indistinguishable from starvation, indistinguishable from death by dangerous medical drugs and pesticides.

Meanwhile, at home, the U.S. AIDS establishment, able to mount a multimillion dollar campaign to make people aware of real immunosuppressive factors, didn't.

No studies of consequence have been done to show what happens when people who are said to have pre-AIDS in America change their immunosuppressive habits. The few fringe efforts in this regard have been ignored, like fleas, at federal health agencies.

It is getting late in the game for the average doctor on the street to plead ignorance.

The cure to what is called AIDS has much to do with the proposition that immune systems can be repaired. Although, in this, medicine has little experience or skill.

In the midst of AIDS deaths, misery, and redefinition, various ideologues who want to purify the world, by their own standards, see big opportunities to attack scapegoats, turn off sex, increase general hatred and expand readiness to allow violence against so-called high-risk groups. They see opportunities to introduce distorted Biblical or medical models of society. What I now want to see are several researcher-prizewinner types, who love to take "human" positions on health matters so earnestly, suddenly step out into the harsh light and blow sirens on the absurd science and bureaucracy of AIDS. Until then, their graduation from the league of baloney slicers is in doubt.

I have dug up some piquant stuff – and of course I am not the first – but now it is these researchers' turn to scour the scene and show in further detail how bizarre, unscientific, afraid, and lying their brethren have been, chapter and verse.

Then the media will cover it.

PART THREE

HIDDEN
IMMUNOSUPPRESSION

CHAPTER TWENTY-FIVE

THE INNER SANCTUM OF THE LABORATORY

I came back again to my anonymous doctor-friend in New York. The central question in our new talks was: Would it be worthwhile to explore various hidden sources of immunosuppression? Sources which ordinarily escape the public eye?

In a sense, that would be like turning around the definition of AIDS on its makers. It would be saying: All right, if you want to define AIDS as virtually all the immunosuppression on the planet, then here are some sources you haven't thought about, don't want to think about, which involve your own home base–science, medical research itself.

The New York doctor suggested I axe this portion of the book.

"People will think it's too weird, too improbable," he said.

After a little thought, I decided to include the following section. Because if AIDS continues to be promoted as a classic infectious plague caused by HIV, one which gobbles up almost every disease symptom known to man, it will obscure other existing sources of ill-health and immune-suppression.

In Africa, for example, chronic long-term starvation will be subsumed under the latest definition of AIDS. AIDS will become the brush that tars the continent, and political realities that make hunger persist will also take a back seat in people's minds. Ordinarily, whenever famine and food-shortfalls strike African countries, there are those local officials who are all too willing to blame Nature exclusively, to stretch toward "natural" explanations.

These officials accept that food already grown within their borders, destined for export back to the industrialized West, cannot be diverted to feed their own people. Not even a fraction of it.

For these officials, as well as for agriculture-multinationals and large local landowners who grow this food, AIDS has an unusual aspect: It explains away hunger, it smokescreens any embarrassment that might be caused by the bizarre juxtaposition of starving people and available food. It calls starvation a viral plague, AIDS.

Likewise, whatever ill-health and death is caused by the sale and dumping of dangerous drugs and pesticides on the Third World, this too can be buried under the idea of AIDS. In fact, new drugs/vaccines can be developed to ship *into* those areas, to treat AIDS.

Let us say I own an airplane hanger full of drums of liquid which will, in exceedingly small amounts, make a person develop fever, vomit, lose weight, walk more slowly, and after months turn a bluish color, asphyxiate and die.

Let us suppose my major concern is marketing this chemical in countries who will allow it to be deployed to kill pests that threaten crops in fields.

Or let us suppose I own a hundred thousand test tubes full of a liquid which will kill human bone marrow, and my major concern is to market this as a product for stopping the progress of a germ.

As chemical aggressions ruin the health of people and kill them, the entity called the immune system is also obviously reduced, mangled and slowed to a halt. Shall we call that war, disease, AIDS, what? Shall we call it bureaucracy, inadvertent malevolence? Does it matter?

There are other, even less visible potential sources of immunosuppression.

Such as the research laboratory itself.

Several independent researchers have looked into apparent outbreaks of what's now been called simian AIDS (SAIDS) at primate research centers around the world, during the 1970s. The National Antivivisection Society of London has published the results of some of these researches. The book is called *Biohazard*, and it is a very interesting look at monkeys, not in the wilds of Africa, but within the wilds of medical research labs. A common practice in that self-contained world is shipping monkeys and their diseased tissue specimens from primate center to primate center – and, in the 70s, this may have contributed to a series of animal disease-outbreaks whose symptoms resembled some of those later listed under the definition of AIDS: diseased lymph nodes, enlarged spleen, opportunistic infections such as staph, pseudomonas, shigella, and wasting away.

Biohazard makes it clear that the passing of monkey-microbes to human handlers can, has, and does happen. There has been ample opportunity to infect handlers and lab workers over the last ten years, and some of this disease could have drifted out into the human populations of cities. Easily.

The staff who researched and wrote *Biohazard* believe that, through frequent injection of an entire catalog of animal and human microbes into monkeys, some germs would have recombined, forming new and possibly virulent disease-agents – for humans.

Monkeys were used during the 1970s war on cancer. In an effort to produce cancer in them so it could be studied, microbes from many species were injected. Monkeys were irradiated, treated with immunosuppressive drugs, in an attempt to weaken them and allow these germs to take hold and do maximum damage and, hopefully, bring about cancers. In this process, as I say, ample opportunity existed for germs from as diverse species as mice and goats to infect, simultaneously, monkey cells, recombine and spawn new germs.

New York's Cold Spring Harbor laboratory has issued two studies of laboratory problems, *Biohazards in Biological Research*, and the *Banbury Report*. They note a number of lab accidents involving animals and the transmission of infection to humans. They also point out that in the worldwide "jungle" of biomedical research labs, where thousands of rooms carry on tens of thousands of experiments, on an ongoing basis, we have a fertile environment for human disease possibilities. These reports make interesting reading.

We need to put imagery aside and realize that laboratories are not temples, and like our nuclear plants, systems of safety are prone to human error. A lab tech who shall remain nameless told me about her days at a major cancer research facility on the east coast. Rooms which should have been sealed, where recombinant viral work was going on, were left open and employees strolled through, picked up their lunches on tables, etc. Her protests to management produced no revisions of habits.

Poorly covered in the U.S., there is an ongoing story of six cases of cancer among lab researchers at the Paris Pasteur Institute (1984-88). These people were all working in two adjoining labs, and the odds of their contracting parallel illnesses have been estimated at 10 million to one.[1] Two of the workers have already died, and finally Pasteur is climbing off its high horse and saying it will investigate the possibilty that the character of the cancer research had something to do with the acquired cancers.

Part of Pasteur Institute's research, it is said, involves implant- ing genes suspected of causing cancer in e-coli bacteria, which are the most common and universal of human bacteria. Could this amount to the creation of several generations of infectious cancer? That is one of the questions Pasteur has apparently been stonewalling.

According to medical activist and author, Jeremy Rifkin, until two years ago safety regulations demanded that bacteria like e-coli be enfeebled, biologically, so that, if they were going to be genetically re- structured, they wouldn't survive long enough to escape lab rooms. That rule, he states, has now been buried, and we are seeing new su- per-strong forms of e-coli used in hazardous bio-research.

The lab is no temple. Michael Gold's book, *A Conspiracy of Cells*, tells the tale of one Henrietta Lack's cervical cancer, which, for over twenty years, was misidentified, ignored, and overloked, as it – in cell culture form (she died in 1951) – contaminated lab experiments from New York to Moscow. Researchers who thought they were do- ing seminal work in liver cancer, work in determining the resistance of normal human cells to radiation, were actually experimenting on Lack's cervical cancer cells, and even today the mess may not be straightened out.

Gold recounts how several of these discredited researchers banded together and tried to discredit in turn the alert bureaucrat who blew the whistle on them – by doctoring photos and essentially con-

---

[1] *American Medical News* July 17, 1987, p.3.

structing an imaginary experiment proving that their work was pure and uncontaminated.

But who would undertake a worldwide probe of lab safety – and possibly discover that many germs exist which, under current practice, could escape into the environment and bring about generations of disease, immunosuppression, and undoubtedly several of the symptoms attributed to AIDS? Why, other scientists, other members of the fraternity.

Would such researchers implicate their own brethren, especially if doing so amounted to professional suicide?

Here is a quote from the book *Biohazard*, which offers a description of monkey experiments conducted at NIH during the 1970s:

"(There was the injection of) various lentiviruses into the brains and bloodstreams of chimpanzees, gibbons, six species of American monkey and eleven species of African or Asian monkey, including the African green . . . Furthermore, in the NIH laboratory, Kuru and CJD viruses have been grown in cultures of African green monkey cells mixed with calf serum and ten other animal viruses. Kuru, CJD, and scrapie have also been injected into goats, cats, guineapigs, skunks, moles, mice, hamsters, rats, ferrets, mink, sheep, opposums, gerbils, and racoons . . . The NIH team was injecting lethal lentiviruses, about which they knew virtually nothing, into a wide range of animals (crossing species-barriers in complex and probably confused patterns). Over a period of twenty years, beginning in 1966, they injected all known forms of lentivirus into African green monkeys, ignorant of the fact that almost half of them (and up to 80% by some estimates) would be carriers of STLV-III, a virus not discovered until 1983 . . . The conclusion is that STLV-III and lentiviruses were given ample opportunity to swap genes . . . and as samples were sent across the world, there were plenty of opportunities for the virus to infect humans."

In essence, many of these monkeys were living test tubes, used to house injected germs from many species. The chance for recombining would be, as the authors say, "ample." What reaction would the new germs have in humans? Unknown.

As for lab accidents, here is a cluster of examples, again from the pages of *Biohazard*:

"Litton (Industries) ran the Frederick Cancer Research Center (Maryland), at which a great deal of basic research was carried out; for this they received government money. However, in 1975 four experiments at Frederick were stopped after the animals became infested with pinworms, and the testing facilities had to be decontaminated. This was due to gaps underneath the doors in laboratories which allowed loose animals to roam from room to room."

Frederick's animal handling procedures were tested in 1976: "A chemical tracer was added to one day's feed for a group of animals. A week later, the tracer was found on walls and floors of the experimental room, in corridors, and on clothing and equipment."[2] Then in September 1977, an epidemic of salmonella[3] occurred among test animals. This incident led to the killing of 51,000 laboratory mice and rats. Epidemics caused by various other viral infections forced Litton to kill a further 89,394 animals in all . . ."

These animals populations at research centers are not small. The centers are regular . . . jungles.

Between 1975 and 1980, *Biohazard* authors report 85 cynomolgus monkeys bit staff at Shamrock Farms, in Sussex. Shamrock is a supplier of primates for lab research. The *Biohazard* authors note that this total doesn't take into account the nine other types of animals held at the facility – and, as to the general microbiological environment we are talking about, the authors cite a 1970s study run by Pfizer, the pharmaceutical house, in which researchers found 140 different viruses in primates and cut off the research, realizing there were more.

The authors reprint a 1983 internal memo of the Maryland SEMA Corporation, which indicates that lab research chimps were being injected with serum from AIDS patients. The chimps had already been exposed to Hepatitis B. In the first month of 1983, three accidents involving monkeys were noted. There is no indication as to

---

[2] RJ Smith, 1979, *Science*, vol. 204, 1287-92.
[3] One of the diseases sufficient for a diagnosis of AIDS.

whether they were the primates who had been exposed to AIDS serum or Hepatitis B:

"1. An animal technician was working with a monkey – the monkey grabbed his glasses – the employee reached into the cage to retrieve his glasses, and the monkey bit him!

"2. A monkey got loose and an animal technician grabbed him with his bare hands – he was bitten.

"3. A procedure involving animal blood from an animal with an undefined condition was being carried out with a punctured glove on a hand with an open cut – and blood got into the cut."

Lawrence Loeb and Kenneth D. Tartof, of the Chase Institute for Cancer Research, in Philadelphia, requested, ten years ago, in a letter to *Science*, (vol. 193, 23 July, 1976) that experiments involving possible cancer-causing viruses cultivated together with primate viruses "be immediately halted until the safety of such experiments are extensively evaluated."

Since a number of animals were developing tumors from a mixed extract of mouse and baboon viruses, the authors feared human contagion. A *British Medical Journal* study (vol. 284, p. 246-8, 23 January, 1982) summarizes accidents among 690 lab staff working at British experimental farms and veterinary centers: 226 injuries in lab accidents and 103 injuries from handling animals.

The *Biohazard* authors categorize accidents from various microorganisms encountered among animals in labs.

Leptospirosis (Bacterial): can produce anything from mild flu to fatal jaundice. Historically, 67 reported cases of accidents. Ten fatal to humans.

Herpes Simian B: Endemic in some monkeys, can be fatal to humans, as a result of brain encephalitis. Seventeen human deaths since 1934. (In 1987, the Pensacola, Florida, Naval Research Center reported three accidents to monkey handlers. As of the summer of 1987, one handler had died, another was in a long-term coma, and a third had recovered. One worker's wife caught the infection from him.)

Strongyloides (Parasite): "In a recent case an animal technician apparently acquired the infection from a primate experimentally inoculated with the parasite at Meloy Laboratories, Springfield, Virginia. This is a round worm parasite which causes chronic diarrhea and intestinal bleeding."

Tuberculosis: The World Health Organization states that monkeys, after cattle, are the most important source of TB infection in humans. Imported primates would constitute the greatest human risk.

Korean Haemorrhagic Fever: At the Korea University Virus Institute in Seoul, between 1971 and 1979, nine cases were reported among people exposed to the virus from rodents.

Hepatitis B: Between 1970 and 1978, 48 lab workers caught the disease from primates worldwide.

Meningitis: "On June 2nd, 1987, *The Guardian* warned that a batch of giant snails imported from Taiwan and Southeast Asia, and destined for school dissection and sale through pet shops, were infected with meningitis."[4]

Biohazard authors, editors, and researchers Jan Creamer, Bill Bingham, Mike Huskisson and Tim Phillips list 20 more microbes that have caused infections in labs. *Biohazard* has not been widely released in the U.S. Its discussions of goings-on in animal labs are potent reading, and not just for people who are convinced of the antivivisection position. Piece by piece, a few accidents here, a few accidents there – one gets the beginnings of an impression as to how large the community of animal labs worldwide really is. That disease could emanate from these facilities begins to seem not at all like science fiction.

Though figures are hard to come by, *Biohazard* authors cite a British Home Office Report stating that, in 1985, 5,869 primates were used in experiments in the U.K. The authors point out that this figure probably does not include defense or public health facilities run by the government. It doesn't include primates killed for tissue for making vaccines, or those used for breeding purposes, or those who die before they can be used in recorded lab experiments.

---

[4] Leptospirosis, strongyloides, tuberculosis, and meningitis could all, by the latest definition, be called AIDS, or pre-AIDS symptoms.

The largest primate supplier in the world is Charles River Research Primates. They own Key Lois island, off Florida, and operate out of six other nations as well. They sell about *22 million lab animals* a year. Worldwide, perhaps 100 million lab animals are killed each year.

Zeroing in on several specific lab practices conveys how easy it is to spread contamination out into the environment, from a business whose economic leader sells 22 million animals a year.

In this regard, *Biohazard* authors reprint a notice from the Oxford University Department of Experimental Psychology primate unit, dated December, 1976: "The standard of hygiene on Level F has recently deteriorated to an aesthetically unpleasant and medically dangerous level . . . The sawdust trays beneath the cages or chairs are not being cleaned out sufficiently often. Last Saturday morning twelve of the trays contained faeces, and presumably urine, together with varying amounts of peanuts, chow, orange peel, banana skin in different stages of fermentation. My attention was drawn to this by a member of the animal staff who was attempting to kill flies attracted by the feast.

"The weighing machine and surrounding floor seem to collect (this kind) of debris . . . Please remember to replace the lid on this bin; it is often left unfastened despite the notice on the lid.

"An animal occasionally urinates or defecates on the floor of a testing room. Please clean it up. There is always a mop and bucket of disinfectant in the cage washing-room.

"Animal hair, urine and faeces are sometimes left in the cage-washing (?) room, where monkeys are anaesthetized. As an experimenter is often the only person who knows that the mess has been deposited, I think we must clean it up ourselves. Finally, the post-mortem room sometimes has dirty instruments, animal hair, etc. This room should be cleaned up as soon as possible after using it."

Stories like this are not rare exceptions, as you'll see if you read various reports issued by independent groups who have managed to do unofficial inspections of animal labs around the world.

Finally, the *Biohazard* authors remark on the shipment of diseased tissue specimens from animal lab to lab. This is SOP. As an example, in the early 80s (and perhaps now) infected baboon brains were shipped from New Guinea to Australian and American labs. They traveled on international commercial airlines twice a week to Holland, where they were transferred to other aircraft and sent to the U.S. It would be foolish to assume that security conditions which are established in labs for diseased specimens (and sometimes don't work) could be consistently maintained via airliners.

A letter sent to the *Lancet*, published on October 11, 1975, illustrates what can happen in related circumstances. Authors AJ Zuckerman and DIH Simpson, of the London School of Hygiene and Tropical Medicine, write the following:

". . . it is only natural that we regularly receive material from all over the world for diagnosis and identification . . . The condition in which many of the specimens arrive causes us extreme concern. Our most recent examples have been badly smashed blood samples sent by post from overseas for hepatitis and Lassa fever studies. These samples were potentially highly infectious, but were so badly packed that serum was leaking freely through the outer paper. There is no need to stress the hazard to postal workers or to those who open the package."

I recently received a "Report on the University of California's Research Facilities," from Peter Hamilton, head of the Lifeforce Foundation in Vancouver, Canada (Box 3117, Main Post Office, Vancouver, BC, Canada, V6B 3X6).

It is the result of a 1982-83, very unofficial inspection of animal labs, and includes photos.

Here are excerpts from his report:

"At one facility, U.C. San Francisco . . . soiled linen was left in hallways, windows of some animals rooms were left open[5] . . . in rooms S1189 and S561, where Herpes and Hepatitis research was being conducted, doors were not sealed properly."

---

[5] Tuberculosis, a common primate disease, is said to be transmissible by airborne routes.

"April 19, 1982. Animal Sciences, University of California at Davis. Hay that was used to feed and house animals was found throughout one public section of hallway, offices and laboratories."

"July, 1982. Fifth Floor, Animal Tower[6], UC San Francisco. Hallway area was found to be extremely cluttered, which would hamper proper sanitation of this area (This was noted on most floors of the Animal Tower.). Garbage and empty fecal trays, etc. were left by the elevator, posing possible health problems for personnel and animals."

"July 27, 1982. Animal Tower, UC San Francisco. Room S589 had cages that had not been properly sanitized for approximately two weeks. The floor in this room had been observed on several occasions to be covered with feces, broken glass from water bottles, etc. In other primate rooms on floors 4, 5 and 6, fecal trays were leaking. Fecal trays that were bent prevented proper disinfecting. Room S400 housed eight monkeys. This room would be difficult to sanitize and the remains of lining that had been removed from the inside of the door left a surface that could not be properly cleaned. This room appears to be a storage room that was not designed to house animals."

"July, 1982. Animal Tower, UC San Francisco. Waste cans did not have lids and leakproof disposable liners. Unemptied containers attracted flies."

"September 17, 1981. June 30, 1982. Warren Hall, Tolman Hall, Life Sciences, Biochemistry, Grizzly Peak, UC Berkeley. Areas were noted with heavy insect infestation; most serious conditions were noted in the basement of Tolman Hall and the fifth floor of Life Sciences."

"July, 1982. Animal Tower, UC San Francisco. There was heavy infestation of cockroaches and flies noted in the cage and bottle cleaning room, in the primate rooms on the 4th, 5th, and 6th floors, in the cat room on the 11th floor and in other areas."

"July, 1982. Animal Tower, UC San Francisco. None of the rooms were sealed, which could cause spread of animal disease to

---

6 This is the Medical Sciences Building, which contains animal research rooms on many of its 14 floors. It also contains human facilities: specialized clinics and diagnostic examining rooms.

other animals, to personnel and to the public. Animal rooms and laboratories were close to or adjoining the (human) hospital."

"July, 1982. UC San Francisco. Soiled (animal) bedding was left in open containers in an outside area near the hospital (human). There was vermin infestation in this area."

"July, 1982. Animal Tower, UC San Francisco. A high infestation of insects was noted in the area used for sanitizing equipment and for storing supplies. This area is located approximately 20 feet from open garbage containers where soiled bedding is placed."

"July, 1982. Animal Tower, UC San Francisco. On the 6th floor, all doors to the animal rooms were unlocked . . . there was a problem with urine falling everywhere except into the fecal pans . . . On the 4th floor, the biohazard room was not sealed. If the ventilation system should stop or lose its efficiency, contamination of the hallway could result."

The researchers who so blithely speculate that AIDS emanated from monekys in Africa have no idea what conditions exist at animal labs around the world, that these labs provide a fertile epidemiological environment for the breeding of contamination and disease. Or if they do have an idea, and some do, they keep their mouths shut.

As pointed out in the medical teaching program, *Nonhuman Primates*, by G.L. Van Hoosier, there are a number of diseases which can be passed from primates to humans. The very fact of catching feral animals in the tropics and bringing them to labs gives you a situation which is "potentially an explosive public health hazard."

Among the bacterial diseases which can potentially move from primates to humans is tuberculosis. In 1972, more than 800 cases of simian TB were reported to the CDC. Other bacterial diseases include enteritis, pneumonia, leptospirosis, and meliodosis. There are several types of enteritis, including salmonellosis, and several pneumonias.

Three protozoan parasites which can move from primates to humans are Entamoeba histolytica and Balantidium coli, both of which cause dysentery in humans; and malaria.

Primates can develop a number of viral infections, among which hepatitis and two types of monkeypox (causing lesions) can be passed to man.

By definition, any of the bacterial infections of primates could be diagnosed as AIDS in humans. The protozoan and viral infections could be easily misdiagnosed in humans and end up looking like one or more AIDS indicator diseases.

Nonhuman Primates stresses the care that must be taken in keeping primate areas in an excellent state of sanitation, in order to help avoid passage of primate disease microorganisms to humans.

I know of no study which has attempted to track animal handlers and animal-lab personnel in, say, the San Francisco area, to see what diseases they have developed and what contact they have had with those subsequently diagnosed with AIDS.

If epidemiologists can command grants which take them to Africa to explore the mysteries of the green monkey, they can take cabs and shuttle flights to major animal labs and start looking for unusual disease there.

A November, 1985, unofficial inspection of Columbia University's animal-research areas by a source who prefers to remain anonymous, brought this summary: "In the Black Building, I saw that food had been thrown into animal cages and fallen into fecal and urine trays. Rooms *stank*. Cages were vertically stacked and urine and feces would spill from top cages to bottom ones. Door marked with signs stating – 'Contagious Diseases, Keep Out' – were unlocked. People in surgical clothes were walking around with dried (animal) blood on their clothes."

To ask a rhetorical question, why doesn't NIH fund a modest study to investigate what diseases animal handlers and lab personnel may have carried into the streets of New York?

In the spring of 1979, about the time AIDS was supposedly percolating, five employees of the University of California School of Medicine came down with Q-fever.[7] One of them died. The source

---

[7] The UC School of Medicine houses the Animal Tower cited often above. Information on this Q-fever outbreak was supplied from articles in *Synapse*,

of the disease was a group of sheep housed on campus in a medical research facility. The state Occupational Safety and Health Administration did an inspection and cited the University for "less than optimal" sanitary conditions.

It turned out that 25 employees in all had been ill with Q-fever during this period. Although university officials tried to downplay the problem, it was the second time such infections had occurred. Ten years, earlier, according to UCSF researcher, Dr. Julius Schacter, "16 percent of the university employees with potential exposure had been infected."

In 1979, the research building where sheep were often transported from their pens was very close to Moffitt Hospital. Sheep sometimes were taken on human passenger elevators.

Other safety violations: Not all employees in the sheep area wore protective garments; those wearing lab coats wore them when they wandered over to the hospital; sheep were sometimes unloaded from their cages, near air in-take systems; sheep and sheep cages were often moved in general university hallways.

Schacter pointed out that, if regulations had been changed after the 1968-9 cluster of Q-fever infections, the same problems wouldn't have arisen ten years later. Peter Hamilton, of the Lifeforce Foundation in Vancouver, recently told me that he still has questions about safety at the UCSF sheep facility. The area does not seem properly contained, he states, and there are no seals on the sheep rooms or negative air pressure to keep microorganisms inside rooms. It is also possible, he feels, that some sheep wastes are being brought over to the waste area of the Animal Tower and dumped in containers about 50-100 feet from Moffitt Hospital. This last possibility needs to be checked further, Hamilton said.

Q-fever can be picked up from feces. It is a rickettsial disease which humans can get from sheep, cattle and goats. Some of the symptoms include acute headache, cough, pneumonitis, abdominal pain, prostration, and fever. The pneumonia occurs in about a third

the UC School of Medicine newspaper, and one of its writers, Charles Piller, who is a well-known science writer.

of the cases on record in the U.S. Less frequently, hepatitis is a complication.

The disease becomes more virulent in those whose immunity is already compromised, judging by several of the people at UCSF who came down with it. They were already in somewhat poor health. Although cases of person-to-person transmission are rare, they have been recorded. The disease has been picked up through breathing the rickettsial organisms, and also from worker's clothing, at a laundry. So the disease-agent is fairly hardy, and can be carried some distance from the original source of infection and remain communicable.

What would Q-fever do, say, in a city like San Francisco, to people who, through massive drug and antibiotic use, already had a number of immune problems?

The answer has not been looked for.

But the symptoms, as usual, all mesh with various definitions of early HIV disease, AIDS, pre-AIDS, and slim.

Acute headache, cough: early HIV disease.

Pneumonitis: AIDS.

Abdominal pain: slim.

Fever: slim, pre-AIDS.

Prostration: slim, pre-AIDS.

Problems with animal facilities at UC San Francisco continued. In March of 1987, a confidential memo concerning conditions at a neurology lab was leaked to the press: "Dead (and in some cases cannibalized) hamsters were observed in a number of cages," the memo said. It also cited problems with an automatic watering system, which soaks down hamsters' cages, and a general failure to monitor the animals.[8]

---

[8] "9 arrested in animal rights protest," by Charles Piller, *Synapse*, April 30, 1987.

CHAPTER TWENTY-SIX

BIOWARFARE RESEARCH

When you suggest that medical facilities, their experimental methods and employees may be contributing to human disease and death, you're going to find a great deal of imagery in your path. Imagery about nice shiny clean labs where nothing could go wrong, imagery that suggests disease escapes from labs only in science-fiction movies. Imagery that shows a strong preference for African jungles as a source of human disease rather than sloppy research rooms.

Introducing the possibility that debilitating disease might come out of biowarfare labs is even more suggestive of science fiction. But, of course, it doesn't take more than a moment's reflection to realize that germs don't mind which sort of facility they're escaping from.

In Europe, the question of whether AIDS could have been made in a lab is much more seriously entertained than in the United States. The U.S. State Department likes to suggest that this is only because Soviet disinformation specialists are madly at work, subverting European newspaper editors. In fact, the questions about chemical/biological warfare (CBW) and AIDS are real enough, and one doesn't have to be a propaganda expert to consider them.

Unfortunately, virtually all those who suggest that AIDS may have come out of a lab buy the principal party line about AIDS, hook, line and sinker. They simply remove the part about the African origin of AIDS and insert the substitution of a lab-altered virus which, in most arguments, turns out to be HIV.

Since there is no evidence that the cases of AIDS being reported around the world are all "the same disease" or from the same source; since there is no evidence that there is a single entity called AIDS; since the listed symptoms of the syndrome can be fulfilled from a number of different sources; since HIV has never been proved to cause human disease . . . there is no reason to assert one has proof that CBW is responsible for "the worldwide plague called AIDS."

However, whether or not CBW research has brought forth germs and chemicals which have caused various forms of immuno-suppression – that is a very reasonable question. It is also very difficult to answer because, to a much greater degree than nuclear science, the types of accidents which have occurred at facilities, and even the types of microbes worked with, are secret.

Nevertheless, since CBW people are massaging microbes with the intent of creating more and more powerful killers, only a fool would cross out the possibility that, on several occasions, they have succeeded to a greater degree than projected. Accidents happen. Intentional experiments also occur, in which human subjects are infected with germs.

99% of the researchers I spoke with while writing this book balked heavily at the suggestion that immunosuppression could have come out of a CBW lab. You would have thought I was implying that Mom had laced one of her apple pies with botulism toxin.

Again, imagery at work. Both professional scientists and the public have been strongly trained to believe that germs for germ warfare actually causing civilian disease is a huge joke only idiots would entertain as potential reality.

This chapter is a short, *very* partial history of CBW incidents. It is culled from very public sources, the *Washington Post,* the *L A Times,* several other newspapers and magazines, and two books: *A Higher Form of Killing* (Paxman and Harris, Hill and Wang publishers, 1982), and *Gene Wars* (Piller and Yamamoto, William Morrow and Company, 1988). In other words, you don't have to get special access to secret files to find out this information.

I am presenting it because I want to establish that, for some time, there have existed people who are willing to use CBW weapons. It is not a fantasy. Since you have read this much of the book, you have inferred by now that many chemicals, particularly those which affect the nervous system, can bring about, among other things, severe weight-loss and wasting away. This, of course, has become a prime symptom of AIDS.

As you read this chronology, you'll notice a number of chemicals. Some of them clearly can do this kind of damage.

Reading this chronology should not only make it clear that some so-called AIDS symptoms can be produced by CBW agents, but that we have a whole industry here which is out of the public view, which has done some very nasty things, which has never been opened for serious government inspection. To say nothing of *public* inspection. In the area of CBW, two very unpleasant strains of human attitude come together: military secrecy and the arrogance of "doctor knows best." They combine to keep in the dark potential effects of laboratory machinations.

On April 22nd, 1915, the Germans used chlorine gas as a military weapon for the first time, in northwest Belgium. By the end of WWI, almost a million deaths and casualties on both sides resulted from the use of chemicals as weapons.

In December, 1947, the Pentagon sent 2 senior biologists from Fort Detrick (center of U.S. biowarfare research) to Japan to look into evidence that germ warfare tests had been carried out there by Japanese General Ishii Shiro. They interviewed a number of Japanese biologists and discovered that what the Japanese had done outstripped Allied research during the second war. The Japanese had worked on anthrax, bubonic plague, tuberculosis, smallpox, typhoid, and cholera. Their records showed that they had deliberately given these germs to prisoners, some of whom died from these diseases.

The General and his associates were granted immunity from prosecution, and Japanese biowarfare specialists were imported and put to work in the U.S., much as Von Braun and his German associates had been given carte blanche in U.S. rocket research, and certain Nazis had been welcomed into what became the CIA.

In 1949, the American Chemical Corps dropped a pint of apparently harmless bacteria into the Pentagon's air conditioning system, to try to map its spread.

Around this time, the U.S. Army also tried to infect four healthy volunteers with huge doses of aerosoled serratia bacteria. They produced only mild symptoms.

In 1950, two U.S. Navy ships sailed up and down around the Golden Gate Bridge and sprayed serratia bacteria for two days on the city of San Francisco. The test was deemed a success because it showed the supposedly harmless bacteria could be spread virtually to every inhabitant of San Francisco. It presumably gave information about what could be done to Americans if the Soviets tried the same sort of attack-pattern. A man recovering from a hernia operation in a San Francisco hospital died of a rare serratia infection. His family sued the federal government and lost. Today, serratia infections are much more common than in 1950.[1]

In 1951, the U.S. Navy contaminated a number of wooden boxes with serratia bacteria, bacillus globigii, and aspergillus fumigatus. They shipped the boxes from a supply depot in Pennsylvania to Norfolk, Va. The Navy wanted to see how easily germs could be spread to people handling the boxes. In particular, they chose aspergillus, according to one report, because they thought black workers would be very prone to catching it.

In 1953, the U.S. Chemical Corps sprayed clouds of bacteria and possibly chemicals (particular ingredients' names not available) over Winnepeg, Canada, and Stony Mountain, Manitoba.

Fort Detrick scientists, in 1950, conducted a number of tests with a crop disease, cereal rust spores. Pigeons were dusted with the spores, flew out 100 miles from their cages, and returned. Tests showed thay had enough spores left to infect the oats in their cages. Some pigeons were then dropped out of planes over the Virgin Islands. Eventually, instead of birds, a bomb was used which released infected turkey feathers.

---

[1] It is also apparent that such experiments helped military scientists determine the feasability of inoculating American populations without their knowledge, against biowarfare agents, via aerosol-vaccines sprayed over cities. Under the AIDS definition's "and other bacterial infections," serratia would today qualify for a diagnosis of AIDS.

In 1953 and 1954, two British operations, Ozone and Negation, used animals strapped to rafts which were floated off the Bahamas. Clouds of bacteria, possibly anthrax and brucella, were released and the animals died. They were burned at sea.

In 1952 or 53, similar British operations were carried out in Europe. These also involved animals, but in cages: mice, guinea-pigs, and rabbits, several thousand in all. They were floated on rafts at sea off Scotland, and also contaminated with clouds of germs. They too died. Their bodies were brought back to shore for analysis.

During the 1950s and 60s, the Utah CBW center, Dugway Proving Ground, in conjunction with the University of Utah, carried on outdoor tests in which animals were infected with Rocky Mountain spotted fever, Q-fever, tularemia, and plague. These tests of dangerous bio-agents were run near populated areas. Apparently the justification used was, the diseases already existed in wild animal populations in the vicinity.

In 1977, it was revealed that the U.S. Army had performed 239 secret biological tests in the U.S. between 1949-1969. Example: In 1965, "biological agents" were spread around at a Greyhound bus terminal in Washington DC. This routine was repeated in 1968 in a New York City subway station.

Meanwhile, by as early as 1953, 1500 British soldiers had been tested for reaction to nerve gases at Porton Down.

Between 1953 and 1957, the U.S. Army handed out $100,000 to the New York Psychiatric Institute, for testing patients' reactions to selected drugs. One of these patients, a tennis pro named Harold Blauer, died after an injection of a mescaline derivative. On May 5, 1987, a New York judge awarded $700,000 to Blauer's estate.

In November of 1953, a senior CIA official named Sid Gottlieb attended a meeting of Fort Detrick scientists and CIA people in the Appalachians. Later, Gottlieb told the men he had put LSD in their drinks. Frank Olson, a civilian scientist from Detrick, arrived home depressed, and a week later jumped to his death from the 10th floor of a New York hotel. Twenty-two years later, Olson's family learned about the LSD connection.

All told, it is estimated that 1500 Armed Forces personnel and civilians were given LSD and other hallucinogens in tests. The figure is clearly understated.

In 1961, Operation Ranch Hand commenced in Vietnam. In the next three years, defoliants were sprayed from Mekong to the DMZ. There were Agents Green, White, Pink, Purple, Blue, and Orange.

During the Vietnam war, Seventh Day Adventists who were serving as non-combatants were exposed to airborne tularemia by Fort Detrick personnel and developed acute tularemia.

At Porton Down, the number one British CBW center, between 1960 and 1966, 33 terminal cancer patients were tested with Langhat Virus and Kyasanur Forest Disease Virus. All the testees died, two after contracting encephalitis.

From the mid-1940s to the mid-1970s, the Manhattan Project, Atomic Energy Commission, and the Energy Research and Development Administration carried out radiation tests on citizens throughout the U.S. In 1945-7, 18 people diagnosed as terminally ill were injected with plutonium. This experiment was run in 4 large hospitals from Tennessee to Northern California.

In 1946-7, six patients with good kidney function were injected with uranium salts at the University of Rochester.

In 1951-2, 14 people were exposed to tritium by breathing, immersion, or ingestion in Richland, Washington.

Radioactive iodine was released deliberately seven times, 1963-5, at the Atomic Energy Commission Reactor Testing station in Idaho. Seven people drank milk from cows that grazed on the contaminated land.

In the early 1960s, 20 elderly people were fed radium or thorium at MIT.

1961-3, 102 people were fed real fallout from Nevada test sites, and simulated particles containing strontium, barium, and cesium, at the University of Chicago and the Argonne National Laboratory.

In the 1960s, 57 normal adults were fed radioactive uranium and manganese spheres at the Los Alamos Scientific Laboratory.

In recent years, there have been several allegations of biowarfare. U.S. intelligence agencies claim an outbreak of anthrax in the Soviet city of Sverdlovsk, in the spring of 1979, was the outcome of a leak from a suspected CBW lab there. Rumor is that 40 to 1000 people died in the incident.

The U.S. states that the Soviet Union has been using yellow fever agent in Afghanistan.

Iran claims Iraq is using mustard gas, and perhaps nerve gas, on Iranian troops. In the fall of 1987, West German police raided 12 companies suspected of shipping Iraq equipment for the production of poison gas.[2]

In several countries where AIDS cases have been reported, allegations of CBW use have been made in the context of wars and revolutions.

1. 1985-6, Angola. UNITA rebels claim they have been attacked by napalm and unidentified chemical agents.

2. According to several accounts, Angola and Mozambique were attacked (1969-74) with unidentified chemical and bio agents by Portugal.

3. An UN report indicates that in 1978 and 1982 South African UNITA rebels attacked Angola with some sort of paralyzing gas. Angola alleges that UNITA, in a later 1984 incident, used an unidentified chemical agent in that war.

4. The USSR states that in 1984, the US, in a Brazilian deforestation program, killed 7000 Indians and caused many birth defects, through the use of chemical herbicides.

In their excellent *A Higher Form of Killing*, Robert Harris and Jeremy Paxman remark that, during the Vietman war, Pentagon people were busy researching blood types on groups of Asians. Were scientists thinking of ways to develop ethnic-specific weapons? Harris and Paxman offer this quote from a Fort Belvoir, Va., 1975 publication, *Decontamination of Water Containing Chemical Warfare Agent*: ". . . it is theoretically possible to develop so-called ethnic chemical weapons, which would be designed to exploit naturally oc-

---

2 The use of chemical weapons in the Iran-Iraq war has now been verified.

curring differences in vulnerability among specific population groups. Thus, such a weapon would be capable of incapacitating or killing a selected enemy population to a significantly greater extent than the population of friendly forces."

Harris and Paxman also offer the comment of a Dr. Leonard MacArthur, in testimony before a 1969 House Appropriations Committee considering budget-funds for defense in the upcoming year: "Within the next 5 to 10 years, it would probably be possible to make a new infective microorganism which could differ in certain important respects from any known disease-causing organisms. Most important of these is that it might be refractory to the immunological and therapeutic processes upon which we depend to maintain our relative freedom from infectious disease."

It appears that Dr. MacArthur is talking about the genetic tailoring of a germ that would directly attack the processes of the immune system.

Paxman and Harris remark that, even as early as 1962, "forty scientists were employed at the US Army biological warfare laboratories on full-time genetics research."

Twenty years ago, Porton Down, the principal British center for CBW research, and its American counterpart, Fort Detrick, cooperated in an experiment to transfer genes between two different strains of plague bacillus. The experiment was successful. By 1988, how far would this sort of research gave gotten?

Statistics are not broadcast widely, but according to Seymour Hersh (*New Republic*, May 6, 1967), Fort Detrick experienced 1218 accidents between 1959 and 1963, including 283 cases of illness from contact with microbes. There were three deaths; in two the cause was anthrax, and the other resulted from exposure to viral equine encephalitis.

"One private Pentagon study," Hersh writes, "listed the top five laboratory diseases at Detrick as tularemia, brucellosis, Q-fever, anthrax and equine encephalitis, in that order."

Hersh notes that another report told of "800 industrial accidents at the Rocky Mountain Arsenal, 10 miles from downtown Denver, where nerve and other gases are produced and stockpiled above ground in metal casks about the size of garbage cans. The production line at the arsenal is immense: more than 150 million gallons of highly toxic waste liquids have been pumped into deep wells, according to the Pentagon."

In 1967, Hersh points up the typical reaction to CBW research from the academic community — which has always been used to carry out individual contracts by the Army, Navy, or CIA. Dean William Stone of the U of Maryland Medical School, which had been doing CBW work for 20 years, said to Hersh, "We only accept work in associated fields of medicine. I don't understand people who feel there is something unethical about any of these studies. We have no feeling we're doing anything unethical or improper."

Such reactions today are also typical. They stem from making certain imaginary distinctions between medical and military research. A contract from the Pentagon may be let out on a germ-agent like brucella. Certain university agriculture departments are already interested in the subject and so they naturally believe there is no harm in doing research for the Army on it. Particularly since funds are available. They don't usually track the future of brucella research and find, for example, that years down the road the CBW establishment might be manufacturing canisters of new and improved brucellosis or developing more powerful aerosol distribution of the germ.

The list of universities that Hersh notes (in 1967) were holding CBW contracts from the Pentagon has not diminished. It has grown longer by 1988, and the money has improved considerably. This, in spite of the fact that Nixon, in 1972, signed a treaty outlawing the production of CBW weapons, as well as banning offensive research on potential bio-agents.

During the last eight years, the official CBW budget has grown to about $100 million a year, and official PR has it that we are only doing defensive research on vaccines, to protect ourselves against possible Soviet attack. In fact, the same sort of arms race exists in this arena as with nuclear weapons. Every defensive strategy can be turned to offensive use, and research on defense is potential research for offense.

In addition, there is now the unresolved question of whether genetic manipulation and the consequent creation of new CBW agents falls under the 1972 treaty – or can we, "in good conscience," assume we never agreed to ban this sort of experimentation? Question or no question, such genetic-recombinant CBW work proceeds in the U.S.

As of 1988, more and more American university scientists are finding that biology's best financial friend is the Pentagon. Money from the National Cancer Institute may be drying up, but the Army still wants work done on vaccines against, say, anthrax – and it's easy to take the money and run, because, the thinking goes, how different is working on this vaccine for the Army than working on it for an agricultural agency?

With funds available for CBW work having quadrupled since 1980, we see a full range of work going on at universities and private corporations throughout America. Some of the projects? Producing genes for the dengue-2 virus, shigella (dysentery), salmonella, and snake venom.

If you consider the CBW category called "basic research," available money moved from about $500,000, in 1981, to $20 million by 1987.

In early 1987, it is reported that the staff of MIT's Biology Department voted to turn down all future funds from the Pentagon for research. After this move, a very nervous university administration said they would cut off the Department's money from *within* MIT. So the MIT biologists folded up their tents and said, all right, we'll accept Pentagon work.

Thomas Mason, a biochemist at the University of Massachusetts, told *Progressive* reporter Seth Shulman that his $1 million dollar Army contract for research on dengue-1 and Japanese encephalitis vaccines was, hopefully, justifiable: "While I may be idealistic, I hope that my research can ultimately lead to a vaccine that could benefit many in the third world who are at risk for these diseases . . . I suppose it is unfortunate that this research is funded by the military. Maybe it should all be funded by civilian agencies . . ."

If only wishing would make it so.

In the November 20, 1987, *Progressive*, Richard Jannaccio, a former science writer for the University of Wisconsin, reported on the University hiring of Philip Sobocinski, a retired Army colonel, "to help professors tailor their research to serve the Pentagon – and bring funding to the school."

Sobocinski had formerly worked at Fort Detrick, where he was deputy commander of the Army Medical Research and Development Command. He oversaw $300 million worth of contracts let out to U.S. Army labs "on five continents."

Jannaccio had originally written the story about this interesting hiring move for the Aug. 24, 1987, *Daily Cardinal*, the University of Wisconsin student newspaper. On August 25th, the University fired him.

What are the chances that an independent scientific group would investigate the CBW industry to see if some of its microbes had been involved in causing any part of what is being called AIDS? The chances would be about zero, just as the chances would be about zero of investigating animal research centers all over the world – without major public pressure.

One interesting example out of the arsenal of biowarfare agents being worked on and utilized in the U.S., is brucella. The canis strain, in humans, has caused the following symptoms in infected laboratory workers: headache, fever, malaise, chills, night sweats, muscular aches and pains in the extremities, pharyngitis and lymphadenopathy. You couldn't get a much better description of what has been call ARC, AIDS-Related Complex, which is listed as a precursor to full-blown AIDS.

Of course, no one is interested in pursuing a lead like brucella. Too many unpleasant ramifications.

Back in the mists of the past (September, 1966), 12 plant physiologists sent a letter to President Johnson protesting the use of defoliant pesticides in Vietnam. An answer was penned by Dixon Donnelley, Assistant Secretary of Defense:

"President Johnson has asked me to reply to your letter. Chemical herbicides are being used in Vietnam to clear jungle growth and reduce the hazards of ambush . . . These chemicals are used extensively in most countries of both the Free World and the Communist Bloc . . . They are not harmful to people, animals, soil or water."

Twenty years later, Vietnam vets managed to win a settlement from U.S. manufacturers for extensive physical damage they had incurred from their exposure to dioxin, a byproduct of the widely sprayed pesticide, Agent Orange. There are advocates who now tie dioxin's immunosuppressive effects to some diagnosed cases of AIDS.

The mainstream press doesn't particularly search out stories like the following, partly because it takes work to get confirmation from several sources, and partly because of the nature of the information: In October of 1985, Mary Jo McConahay, representing the Pacific News Service, spoke with a Salvadoran doctor who had lived in Guazapa before being captured by the Salvadoran Army. Dr. Miguel Orellana told her that since January of 1985, " . . . my campaneros and I have started to detect a series of sicknesses which have never appeared in the (Guazapa) zone before. It's an epidemic of something like hepatitis. Its symptoms include serious explosive diarrhea. It must be a viral diarrhea.[3]   Salvadoran children have diarrhea all the time but don't die. But in this type of diarrhea, which is accompanied by skin problems, the children are dying. And in the adult there is extreme physical weakness. When the Salvadoran peasant has malaria he walks and works, but with this he doesn't. He fades, grows weaker and weaker. He passes eight to 10 days with pain in his bones and a strong fever. In the January (military) operation in the zones of Mirandilla and Las Pavas, the people noted something unusual: the bombs weren't the same color as smoke, but rather gray. They exploded differently. One or two weeks later the first cases appeared in Mirandilla, Las Pavas, El Salitre, and it spread."[4]

From time to time, various scenarios having to do with biological warfare surface, and these are written off. In the mid 1960s, MIT professor Salvador Luria raised a few eyebrows when he expressed concern, not optimism, about the "dangers that genetic surgery, once

---

[3] Agents of viral diarrhea have been tested on inmates at US prisons.

[4] Reported by James Ridgeway in the *Village Voice*, Dec. 3, 1985.

it becomes feasible, can create if misapplied." Luria pointed out that fruit flies could be infected with a virus which then changes their metabolisms so they suddenly become oversensitized to carbon dioxide. CO_2 becomes a lethal poison for them.

In the same way, Luria suggests[5] , human populations could be seeded with viruses, making them susceptible to introduced chemicals which, ordinarily, would have no effect, but would quickly become lethal.

Indicating that as of 1987, 127 sites around the U.S. were doing CBW research, including universities, foundations, and private corporations, a *Science* report (Feb. 27, 1987) stated: "The Department of Defense is applying recombinant DNA techniques (genetic engineering) in research and the production of a range of pathogens and toxins, including botulism, anthrax, and yellow fever."

In a speech given at a NY Lenox Hill Hospital AIDS symposium, on April 10, 1983, US Representative Ted Weiss, like Salvador Luria of MIT, raised a few eyebrows when he offered this piece of advice: ". . . as far fetched as it may seem, given the attitudes toward homosexuals and homosexuality by some segments of society, the possible utilization of biological weapons must be seriously explored." Presumably, Weiss was serious about recommending an investigation, but no consensus yet exists for opening up the subject in earnest.

Even the medical community has occasionally expressed doubts about the implications of genetically engineered germs. Twenty years ago in the *Lancet*, Nobel prize-winner FM Burnet commented: "Any escape into circulation (of lab-altered viruses) that was not immediately dealt with could grow into the most unimaginable virgin-soil epidemic . . . involving all the populous regions of the world."

In 1985, the prestigious Cold Spring Harbor *Banbury Report*, undertaken in part of because of nervousness within the scientific community about genetic engineering, made the following speculations under a heading, WORST CASE SCENARIO: DESIGN FOR A

---

[5] See *Biological Time Bomb*, by Gordon Rattray Taylor, World Publishing, 1968.

MAXIMALLY MALIGNANT MONSTER VIRUS: "Because we know the primary structure of many viral genes and have the technical capacity to synthesize both genes and gene products, it would appear that the planned design of either friendly or unfriendly viruses is not too remote a possibility. If the latter should be the perverse goal of our paranoid society, can we construct a virus worse than rabies virus with its 100% case fatality rate or influenza virus with its pandemic potential for 20 million deaths worldwide? In hypothetical phenotype, yes." The authors then go on to list a number of other characteristics of this monster germ and conclude that, in toto, the creation of it would defy "the macabre skills of Dr. Frankenstein himself."

Then, under a small section headed, "The Extended Environment," the authors discuss "the unexplained appearance of a genetically unaltered 1951 influenza virus in 1977 . . . (it has) reminded us that our freezers are potential if unlikely sources of 'new' pathogens." The 1951 virus — flu being notorious for its fast mutation rate — had not changed in 26 years. So it must have escaped in 1977 from a lab freezer.

The authors go on to concede that it is foolish to ignore the present-day Collective Laboratory, with its thousands and thousands of rooms, internationally, as a source for discovery of germs causing disease.

Robert Lederer, in his 1987 article in *Covert Action Information Bulletin* Number 28, "Precedents for AIDS?", summarizes a series of tests on prisoners which could rightly be called biowarfare: "From 1965 to 1968, 70 prisoners, mostly black, at Holmesburg State Prison in Philadelphia, were the subjects of tests by Dow Chemical Company of the effects of dioxin, the highly toxic chemical contaminant of Agent Orange. Their skins were deliberately exposed to large doses and then monitored to watch the results. According to the doctor in charge, Albert Kligman, a University of Pennsylvania dermatologist, several subjects developed lesions which 'lasted for four to seven months, since no effort was made to speed healing by active treatment.' At a 1980 federal Environmental Protection Agency hearing where the experiments came to light, Kligman testified that no follow-up was done on subjects for possible development of cancer.

This was the second such experiment commissioned by Dow, the previous one carried out on 51 'volunteers,' believed also to have been prisoners."

In Vietnam, aside from the dioxin-containing Agent Orange, the U.S. Army employed what was called "a short-term incapacitant," CS (orthochlorobenzamalonitrile). A powder disseminated into the air by grenades, bombs, and shells, it causes intense pain in the upper respiratory tract, severe skin-blistering in humid weather, and brings on acute anxiety and feelings of suffocation.

In 1965, the U.S. Army ordered 253,000 pounds for use in Vietnam. By 1969, the annual demand was up to 6 *million* pounds.

In WWI, civilians accounted for 5% of total fatalities. In WWII, that figure jumped to 48%. In Korea, it was 84%. Vietnam or Afghanistan would certainly rank with Korea. The kind of warfare-development implied by these figures dovetails with a mentality that would, as a matter of course, order 6 million pounds of an incapacitant for a year's use.

Let's sweep away the social knee-jerk reaction to biowarfare scenarios. People bluster and rave about paranoid conspiratorialists and so forth. And yes, there *are* certainly people who interpret breakfast or doing their laundry as directed from the Kremlin or Venus. It doesn't follow, as day from night, that waging limited CBW or carrying out CBW experiments is probability-zero. Not at all.

This is important, because a wholly unwarranted defense of the purity of medical and biowarfare laboratories has taken place based on knee-jerking.

The contemplation of possible numbers alone is sobering. How many germs are being dealt with by how many humans in how many labs in how many countries in how many experiments every day of every year around the world? Have you ever prowled through the stacks of a good biomedical library and gazed at the cumulative published results of this worldwide activity?

The chances really are that many, many microbes have wended their way out of labs into the ordinary environment in which we live; and this is just to talk about *accidental* spreading of germs.

The ex-PR chief of Lawrence Livermore Labs, Bill Perry, once told me in an interview, "I would walk over to the office of a man doing research on nuclear weapons, and I'd ask him how it was going today and he'd sigh and say, 'If I could only get more grant money,' and then I'd tell him, 'Look — with another few million dollars you couldn't do any more than blow up the world two extra times.' He'd say, 'Oh no, you don't understand. This is a *physics* problem.'"

And those are the nice guys.

In 1977 Senate hearings held by the Subcommittee on Health and Scientific Research, a U.S. Army report noted that "the advent of limited war and small scale conflict evoked a need for weapons which could assist in controlling conflict with minimum casualties."

Had the biowarfare research community been working on such weapons, particularly for use in the nonwhite Third World?

In the November 1970 issue of *Military Review,* geneticist Carl Larson pointed out the possibility of designing chemicals to attack specific populations. Larson felt that "observed variations in drug response have pointed to the possibility of great innate differences in vulnerability to chemical agents between different populations."

How far from CBW is it when patients with minimal symptoms are given dangerous pharmaceuticals? When patients with no symptoms are, in effect, being handed death sentences?

I recently spoke with an AIDS clinician who sees patients on referral from other physicians. He is usually able to spot trends in diagnosis before they become widely known.

He told me that the patients who are now coming into his office have weirder and weirder stories. Some are being diagnosed as having full-blown AIDS because of a positive HIV test when they have no symptoms.

One patient was told he had AIDS only because of a blood test which measured the numbers of his T-cells. It was slightly below normal. He had no symptoms, but he was gay. It seemed that this last was the deciding factor.

Another patient was diagnosed as having AIDS by an ophthalmologist, because he was gay and had conjunctivitis in one eye. No HIV test. No nothing.

"Patients," the clinician told me, "seem less educated than ever. They just automatically assume that when the doctor tells them they have AIDS, they have it. Symptoms aren't important. Blood tests aren't important."

A woman who tested positive for HIV but had no symptoms was sold by her doctor on entering an AZT study. This despite the fact that her numbers of immune T-cells were very high,[6] indicating that her immune response was good.

A man in California was likewise convinced by his doctor to enter an AZT study, even though he too had no symptoms. The man was high- pressured. He was told that AZT could extend a patient's lifespan four years. Not only has this never been proven, but AZT itself hasn't been around as an AIDS medication for four years!

---

[6] The count was 1000.

CHAPTER TWENTY-SEVEN

HOW MUCH OF AIDS IS SYPHILIS? AN INTERVIEW WITH DR. STEPHEN CAIAZZA

A flurry of articles has appeared on AIDS as syphilis in the past year. As usual, many supporters of this idea automatically assume that there is one unified disease-entity called AIDS which, instead of being caused by HIV, is caused by the syphilis spirochete.

However, the work of Dr. Caiazza in treating patients diagnosed with AIDS indicates that here is a testable hypothesis. His case records show his patients are recovering. His work could be tested, replicated, or challenged by other physicians.

So far, however, NIH shows no interest in expending the negligible amounts of money it would take to do that job.

At any rate, recent skyrocketing statistics of new syphilis cases in the US have caught medical attention.[1]

Several researchers assert the following:

1) Much syphilis today goes unnoticed, or is misdiagnosed as other disease – possibly AIDS.

2) Syphilis is often treated with inadequate doses of penicillin.

Doctors Klaus Dierig, Urban Waldthaler, and Stephen Caiazza have reported encouraging results in handling AIDS patients with extensive programs of penicillin and other antibiotics.

3) Disproportionately large numbers of syphilis cases, in the last ten years, have occurred in the U.S. male gay and IV drug-user populations.[2]

4) The dementia associated with AIDS may be late-stage neurosyphilis.

---

[1] *The Atlantic* January, 1988, "AIDS and Syphilis," Katie Leishman.
[2] Ibid.

5) There is an overlap of symptoms between AIDS and syphilis, including generalized lymphadenopathy, which is one of the signs of secondary syphilis, skin rashes, weight-loss, fever, sore throat, malaise, sweating, cranial nerve problems, opportunistic infections like candida. And on the whole, both AIDS and syphilis affect more males than females. (Of course, many diseases overlap symptoms with what is called AIDS.)[3]

Venereal disease would not be a popular interpretation of AIDS symptoms. No novelty in a discovery like this. There is no quick tie-in to research on new drugs or new vaccines. There is only better management of penicillin. There are no Nobels waiting for the man who says, "Look for syphilis in your AIDS patients."

Nitrite inhalants may rank at the top of the list of relevant factors in Kaposi's sarcoma, but syphilis may be involved, too. As Harris Coulter points out in his book, *AIDS and Syphilis, the Hidden Link* (North Atlantic Books, Berkeley, 1987), Kaposi's and syphilis share certain traits: ear lesions of a purple color, lung gummata, sarcoid-like granulomas, and strawberry facial lesions.

In addition, older medical literature indicates a potential overlap between syphilitic pneumonia and pneumocystis pneumonia in people with syphilis.

Sporadic studies have indicated high rates of syphilis in Ruanda, northeastern Zaire, and Uganda, areas in which AIDS is reported. This, taken together with accounts of syphilis in Haiti, and, as mentioned, syphilis in the US IV-drug and male-gay populations, could explain the puzzling geographic distribution of some diagnosed AIDS cases.

Coulter concludes that the disappearance of syphilis in the U.S. during the 1950s was achieved "by antibiotic abuse, suppressing the disease (instead of knocking it out) and causing it to smoulder away like an underground fire. It has slowly burned out the immune systems of a large proportion of those who have been (poorly) treated".

---

[3] Several animal studies indicate that syphilis depressed T-cells and macrophages, and also shrank the thymus gland (where T-cells are made). DR Tabor, *Immunology*, Sep. 1987, v. 62, p. 127; O Bagasra, *Immunology*, Sep. 1985, v. 56, p. 9.

Coulter quotes Dr. Armand J. Pereyra ("A Graphic Guide for Clinical Management of Latent Syphilis," California Medicine, 112:5 (1970)):

"Although the incidence of (syphilis) has more than trebled since 1955, the chancre and the secondary rash no longer are commonly seen. Undoubtedly some of these lesions are being suppressed, and the disease masked by the indiscriminate use of antibiotics. It is difficult otherwise to explain the predominance of latent syphilis in current medical practice. The ominous prospect of a widespread resurgence of the disease in its tertiary form looms ahead."

Dr. Stephen Caiazza, a New York physician, has been treating AIDS patients for syphilis. For the past year, he has combined a regimen of penicillin and doxycycline, and out of 125-50 patients, he reports only one has died.

I interviewed him on March 21, 1988.

Q: Originally, you were using IV penicillin for 20-30 consecutive days. What changed your approach?

A: Several things. You can't put everybody in the hospital for the IV. I also found that the most important factor, beyond quantity of medication, was duration of treatment.

Q: So you don't stop.

A: These 125 patients are all still receiving doxycycline, some after a year. I have no idea how long that will have to continue.

Q: What made you originally suspect that some people diagnosed with AIDS actually had syphilis?

A: I wasn't seeing any syphilis in my gay patients. I was treating them for every other kind of STD. So I said, where is the syphilis?

Q: The tests weren't showing it.

A: The tests are totally inadequate.

I started two AIDS patients on a penicillin treatment for syphilis. Their AIDS got better, and when I stopped the treatment, they died.

What I learned from several trips to Poland, where they do a much better job than we do with syphilis, is that the longer a patient has the syphilis spirochetes, the longer it takes them to produce the next generation of spirochetes. That means you have to stretch out the treatment, or you will miss the moment when you can attack the organisms, when they are vulnerable (when they are reproducing).

Q: Your patients – these 125 – are really better?

A: Absolutely. By bloodwork and by clinical symptoms. We naturally watch both factors. They become able to work, to come to the office unassisted and to do things that require energy. Their T and B-cells improve too, slowly, but they improve.

Q: The doxycycline can cross the blood-brain barrier and get to these spirochetes that exist in the brain?

A: Yes, the drug does that.

Q: Is this your only treatment, the penicillin and then the doxycycline?

A: Nutrition is very important. If the patient isn't getting what he needs, the drugs aren't going to work. For example, let's say he had been doing poppers. That binds up vitamin B-12, so he can't utilize it. In that case, his immune system just isn't going to produce. We do complete case histories on our patients.

Q: You can do this treatment, at first with penicillin, by injection in your office?

A: Yes. Once a week. Eventually, when we start doing the doxycycline, that is orally administered. The patient starts out with 400 milligrams a day, 200 twice. Eventually, we halve that dose. But the beginning of treatment is a period of intramuscular injected penicillin.

Q: Are there other physicians in the U.S. who are replicating your results with their patients?

A: None have been doing it long enough, but I'm happy to say a few are starting out with this regimen. I'm getting a grass roots response from doctors and patients. We recently went down to Miami and gave a talk to both doctors and patients there, which went very well.

Q: What has been the response of "health authorities?"

A: Zero. I've talked to a number of officials in New York, both city and state, and they aren't interested at all.

Q: Are they trying to stop you?

A: They can't. Since I'm a licensed physician, I can prescribe penicillin. That part is simple. But I am involved in another legal matter with New York State. A completely unrelated matter, if you get my drift.

Q: And what about the CDC and NIH?

A: Are you kidding? All the research money that's available for AIDS is going to the retrovirologists. That isn't really a great deal of money. But whatever there is, is controlled by Bob Gallo, who is the chief retrovirologist on AIDS research. Now if he's right, he'll get the Nobel prize. And if he's right, he deserves it. But if I'm right, he'll have to unpack his bags for Stockholm. So do you think I'm going to get any money to expand my work on syphilis?

Q: Prior to treating your AIDS patients for syphilis, what were you doing?

A: From 1983 to 1986, I was just another doctor handling AIDS cases, doing the usual treatments, the best ones that were available. Many of those people died. About one a *week*. Now, in the last year, one has died. I mean, *I* can't believe it.

Q: Obviously, there would be no economic payoff for the medical industry if your approach were to win out.

A: Certainly not for the pharmaceutical houses. This treatment is cheap. And syphilis is a boring, prosaic disease. Not much excitement there for researchers.

Q: Once again, these 125 patients of yours. They all have been diagnosed as having AIDS? Are some just HIV-positive?

A: They are either full-blown AIDS cases, or people who have been told they have ARC (pre-AIDS).

Q: The majority of your AIDS patients have had which infections? Pneumocystis?

A: Pneumocystis and/or Kaposi's sarcoma. About 10% were diagnosed with AIDS for other infections.

CHAPTER TWENTY-EIGHT

AFRICAN SWINE FEVER, FIDEL, AND THE CIA

This is another case of a disease which has gotten short shrift in the AIDS research community despite early interest.

The story behind it is quite unusual.

What follows is an article I wrote that was originally published (in a slightly different form) in the *San Jose Metro* on June 4th, 1987. The first paragraphs are concerned with the green monkey theory. I've left them in so you can see that as early as May 1987, U.S. federal health agencies were throwing up their hands in futility about this widely accepted version of how AIDS came to be. Here and there in this article, written at the beginning of my investigation on AIDS, it will be implied that HIV is the cause of one disease-entity called AIDS. We've already covered those unproven creative beliefs.

Where did AIDS come from?

The Surgeon General's office in Washington referred me to the National Cancer Institute. NCI told me that this matter of origins was possibly "a Harvard question."

The Centers for Disease Control (CDC) in Atlanta said, "There is no official version. We're not in very deep on that."

At the National Institutes of Health, I spoke with Don Robusky in Public Affairs. He said, "The accepted wisdom on the origin of AIDS is the green monkey (African). But nobody's really sure . . . The more we find out about that goddamn HIV virus the more devilish and diabolical it becomes."

The National Institute of Allergy and Infectious Diseases: "(Chief of Research) Anthony Fauci here thinks it's Africa, but he's not sure how the virus crossed over from animal to man. There is speculation that Africans ate a green monkey and caught the virus. They do eat monkeys."

The National Academy of Sciences: "It might be the spider monkey. Researchers don't seem to know how it was transmitted from monkey to man."

Dr. Jacques Leibowitch, early French researcher on the disease, consulting immunologist for the World Health Organization, and author of *A Strange Virus of Unknown Origin* (Ballantine): "Who at (the) period (1974-7) could have opened the Zaire jungles or those of neighboring countries and spread the hidden virus in this fashion . . . The Cubans, perhaps. After all, did they not physically intervene in Angola in 1972 . . . Carried by such veterans, (an animal) virus might have pursued its long journey in the direction of the United States. In 1977-8, the Cuban government expelled a certain number of undesirables among whom figured "magalitas" (homosexuals) and Angola veterans. A certain number of the latter found refuge in Florida, in Miami . . . Thus might have been born a new epidemic, out of the jungle depths of Africa into the Western world."

On the matter of the African virus-transference, or jumping of species, there are several scenarios:

Some of the hundreds of types of jungle insects bit green monkeys, then bit humans, passing along the virus.

Humans killed monkeys and monkey blood washed through human sores or cuts.

Humans ate monkeys.

But Dr. James Mullins, Harvard researcher, cautioned in a telephone converstation: "The monkey virus in question is not the AIDS virus. It's the closest we've found to the disease, along with another virus we've discovered in West Africans. But these viruses aren't even close (structurally) to AIDS.

"Eating an infected (green) monkey isn't going to result in anybody getting AIDS. . ."

There have been suggestions that a virus other than HIV is involved. African Swine Fever (ASF).

In 1971 and 1980, Cuba suffered epidemics of ASF. Press coverage in the *San Francisco Chronicle* and *Newsday*, and by Jack Anderson, as well as references in William Blum's *The CIA, Its Forgotten History*, trace possible CIA involvement in the 1971 epidemic. In this scenario, Swine Fever germs were exported from the U.S., possibly through Haiti, into Cuba, as part of the CIA's ongoing revenge-program against Fidel Castro. 500,000 pigs in Cuba consequently had to be destroyed to prevent further spread of the disease. Cuban officials at the time concluded that Cuban citizens were also contracting the Swine Fever in the form of backbreak fever, which in some cases was fatal.

John Stockwell, former CIA station chief in Angola, and veteran Agency watcher, confirms a "90% certainty that this CIA program of Cuban-pig infestation took place in 1971."

The possibility also exists (see, for example, Blum's *CIA*) of other CIA dirty tricks of the period: infecting Cuban turkeys, destroying sugar cane crops, etc.

The original story linking ASF and Cuba and the CIA was written by Drew Fetherston and John Cummings. It was published on January 9,1977, in *Newsday*. The story began:

"With at least the tacit backing of U.S. Central Intelligence Agency officials, operatives linked to anti-Castro terrorists introduced African swine fever virus into Cuba in 1971. Six weeks later an outbreak of the disease forced the slaughter of 500,000 pigs to prevent a nationwide animal epidemic.

"A U.S. intelligence source told *Newsday* he was given the virus in a sealed, unmarked container at a U.S. Army base and CIA training ground in the Panama Canal Zone, with instructions to turn it over to the anti-Castro group."

Fetherston and Cummings, over a period of four months, had interviewed various U.S. intelligence sources and Cuban exiles, in order to piece together a scenario. Their primary U.S. intelligence source said that he had been given the container of ASFV[1] at Fort Gulick, in the panama Canal Zone. Gulick is also the location, it is said, of a CIA training center for mercenaries and career agency people.

---

[1] African Swine Fever Virus.

The container of ASFV ended up on a boat, a fishing trawler off the coast of Panama near Bocas Del Toro. Next stop, Navassa Island, between Haiti and Jamaica. In March 1971, the container arrived in Cuba near the U.S. naval base, Guantanamo.

The first sick Cuban pigs were discovered in early May.

As to whether the second 1980 outbreak of ASF in Cuba was a result of a gift from the CIA, a Cuban national, Eduardo Perez, on trial in New York Federal District Court, on September 10, 1984, testified that in 1980, as part of a biological warfare scheme against the Castro Cuban economy, "a ship traveled from Florida to Cuba with germs..."

Perez indicates the germs inadvertently infected Cuban exiles. And in June, 1980, Peter Winn, in *The Nation*, provided this piece of suggestive background: "During the past two years, Cuba has seen plant blights decimate its sugar, tobacco, and coffee crops, swine fever destroy its hog herds, and a Greek tanker foul its shellfish beds. This simultaneous destruction of Cuba's major foreign exchange-earners and most important meat source has no parallel in Cuban history."

All coincidence?

The AIDS trail which Jacques Leibowitch traces, from Cuba, by boatloads, to Miami, could instead have contained gay men who were infected with the CIA's Swine Fever. A "return gift."

In 1983, two Boston scientists, John Beldekas (Boston University School of Medicine) and Jane Teas (Havard School of Public Health), wondered whether ASF was, in fact, the AIDS virus researchers should be investigating.

They found evidence that ASF was showing up in the blood of AIDS patients, "even though Swine Fever isn't supposed to infect humans," Beldekas comments. This blood-finding sparked a 1986 row with the CDC.

After much arm-twisting, the CDC ran their own tests, claimed Teas and Beldekas were wrong, had make mistakes, and there was no ASF in the blood of those AIDS patients.

Teas traveled to Florida. "There I heard rumors," she recalls, "that some Haitians, after eating pork, were contracting an odd illness . . . Regardless, it was already clear that in some areas where you saw a concentration of AIDS (Africa, Brazil, Haiti), you saw outbreaks of Swine Fever in herds of pigs. Although the pork industry and government scientists won't admit it, there are ASF-infected wild pigs in Florida."

The U.S. Dept. of Agriculture (USDA) disputes this. Teas claims the USDA finally tested a small batch of south Florida pigs and found one that had ASF. USDA sources claim they have no record of the test.

In a July, 1986, letter to the *NY Times*, Douglas Feldman, a medical anthropologist at Yale, registered his own surprise on the subject of ASF:

"Last September, while conducting a preliminary sociomedical study on acquired immune deficiency syndrome (AIDS) in Rwanda, in the eastern part of Central Africa, I was surprised to learn that 50% of the pig population had died in an African swine fever epidemic that had begun in December 1983. The epidemic spread northward from Burundi to south-central Rwanda near Butare . . . with the recent African swine fever scare caused by the discovery of sickly pigs near Belle Glade, Florida, and with the report by Dr. John Beldekas of Boston University and his associates of some evidence of infection by the African swine fever virus in nearly half of a sample of 21 AIDS patients in the United States, epidemiologists and veterinarians might do well to explore the possibility that this virus is a co-factor in AIDS transmission in central Africa and perhaps other regions of the world."

To date, no such exploratory study has been undertaken.

Teas states at least two human studies have shown that ASF can be contracted by humans: "One was done at the US Department of Agriculture's Plum Island facility off Long Island, where exotic animal diseases, like ASF, are studied. They examined 47 staff, and 6 tested positive for ASF. Then another test was run, and they said the first test was incorrect and no one was infected with ASF.

"There is also a New York Health Department study of healthy blood donors which showed that five people had the standard signs of ASF in their blood."

In September 1985, the New York City Health Department did test 160 random blood donors at the New York Blood Center for evidence of Swine Fever. Five showed signs of having contacted the virus. This is quite remarkable, since the prevailing wisdom on African Swine Fever is that humans can't catch it.

Yet instead of trumpeting the finding, the NYC Health Department chose to emphasize that their results didn't justify linking AIDS to Swine Fever. Surely, the confirmed finding of humans with evidence of ASF in their blood should have provoked more studies. None were done.

Beldekas points out how difficult it can be to get an OK to test for the presence of viruses, like ASF, in blood. "To run the lab tests, you need reagents (certain proteins), and these are controlled rigidly by the major research centers. They won't release them to you. This is their way of controlling what research lines can and can't be explored."

Needless to say, the billion-dollar pork industry would be disturbed at charges that:

1. There is a trace of Swine Fever among hogs in the U.S.
2. ASF might be connected with AIDS.
3. AIDS might be contracted from eating pork

Teas: "When ASF swept Brazil in 1978, public pork consumption dropped 30% overnight because of the scare" – regardless of claims that the diseased hogs were being destroyed and that humans could not catch the infection.

There is, according to Teas, much scientific debate about the action of ASF viruses on immune-cells. Depending on which strain of ASF (Portugese or Ugandan) is used in lab tests, it may look like ASF is a cell proliferator (cancer) or a cell-destroyer (AIDS).

I spoke with William Hess, a researcher of exotic animal diseases at the US Dept. of Agriculture's Plum Island facility in New York. Hess, called "the grand old man of Swine Fever," maintained that "there is no evidence ASF can infect humans." He also stated that if the charge against the CIA, re Cuban pig-infection in 1971, is true, "The Swine Fever couldn't have come from Plum Island. We didn't have the virus then."

Then Hess volunteered a remarkable development. Robert Gallo, the number one American researcher on AIDS, at the National Cancer Institute, had recently ordered and been sent a "(viral) probe of ASF for study."

If Gallo is now considering Swine Fever as AIDS-related, he will be the first famous AIDS researcher to step out on dangerous political ice.

Jane Teas adjusts the scenario of Cuban gays, possibly infected with ASF, coming over on the boatloads to Miami: "There were wild pigs, infected with ASF, which were brought to Florida on both Cuban and Haitian boatlifts."

It remains to be seen whether a connection between AIDS and Swine Fever will be explored at NIH. Any positive pronouncements on such a connection would cause a mighty uproar, rekindling the old scenario of CIA-Cuba dirty tricks, dragging the Ameican pork industry into it, and raising the question of why it took so long to heed the work of Beldekas, Teas and others.

African Swine Fever, in pigs, can produce pneumonia, swollen lymph nodes, slow wasting away, skin lesions, and of course fever. There are also brain complications.

Several interesting factors concerning ASF are mentioned by Robert Lederer in his article, "Origin and Spread of AIDS: Is the West Responsible" (*Covert Action Information Bulletin,* Issue 29, Winter 1988). Hog cholera, a disease with the same symptoms as ASF, was attacked by the development of a vaccine, in the 1960s – but the vaccine unfortunately seemed to have been manufactured from pig blood which contained ASFV. "Thus," Lederer suggests, "during mass (pig) vaccination programs, the tainted vaccine prevented hog cholera but also *induced* ASF on a mass scale."

Ben Dupuy, editor of New York's *Haiti Progress,* told Lederer he believes the hog cholera vaccine was intentionally introduced into Haiti to blast the poor-peasant infrastructure. With the death of their pigs during the ensuing ASF epidemic of 1979, Dupuy maintains peasants were forced to pay $100 apiece for new pigs brought in from the U.S. Of course, they couldn't afford this. The idea was to drive peasants off their land into low-paying urban jobs and, from the outside, establish a new U.S.-controlled Haitian economy of huge farms and factories.

In this regard, Lederer also cites an article from the *New York Native*, Dec. 17, 1984, in which Jane Teas remarks that ASF first broke out in Haiti in a well-populated valley that was due to be flooded, as part of a hydroelectric dam project.

John Beldekas told Jack Anderson and Dale Van Atta (*Washington Post*, Oct. 7, 1985) that after he had found signs of ASF in the blood of people diagnosed with AIDS, U.S. Dept. of Agriculture officials told him to keep his mouth shut about it, "for national security reasons . . ."

Two other aspects of ASF are worth mentioning. According to one report, the mariel Cuban boatlift to Florida, during the Carter administration, was at least one-third gay. Apparently, the Cuban government, which is anti-gay, had spy squads searching out and reporting on gay activity in Cuba, and had sent some of these gay men to the U.S. Several thousand were sponsored in the U.S. through gay groups, and the major number of these men ended up in New York, LA, and San Francisco, the three cities where AIDS cases have been reported in large numbers.

It is speculated that some of these men were suffering from ASF. They eventually became active on the bathhouse scene.

Finally, another word on the economic pressure that would surround a public disclosure that ASF was present in animals in the U.S. The following attribution to the U.S. Dept. of Agriculture (1981 pamphlet) was made in the *New York Native* on June 2, 1985:

"On the export side, if African Swine Fever Virus became established in the U.S., there would be an annual loss of some 300 million dollars in pork and related products, plus a partial or complete embargo on other U.S. agricultural exports, including grain, soy beans, and cotton, which now total $25 billion annually."

CHAPTER TWENTY-NINE

CMV (CYTOMEGALOVIRUS)

Before the announcement, in 1984, that HIV was the cause of AIDS, there was considerable give-and-take in medical journals as researchers looked for relevant AIDS factors. One of those cited most often, CMV, disappeared as a possible cause after 1984. It's worth resurrecting a little of that literature.

First, a few researchers spuriously reject CMV because, they say, it has been around for awhile and AIDS hasn't. We have already dealt with this argument in another form, but there are two other rejoinders in the case of CMV: 1) Indications are that, at least among the U.S. male gay population, people are being infected repetitively, by different strains of CMV, as a result of many sexual contacts. This could change the effect of the virus in the body, from former years. 2) CMV working in concert with cofactors, like poppers and other drugs, could exert again, a more harmful effect than usual.

In the *Annals of the NY Academy of Sciences* (vol. 437, p. 320-4, 1984) Lawrence Drew and Lawrence Mintz examine CMV. They note that CMV "is known to cause T-cell dysfunction during acute infectious mononucleosis-like infection," and that of 164 AIDS patients "tested by the CDC for CMV antibody, 162 were positive."

Drew and Mintz tested 56 patients with Kaposi's sarcoma and found all 56 were positive for CMV. They concluded, ". . . we feel that the evidence is compelling that the virus makes a very substantial contribution to the development of Kaposi's sarcoma."

Martin Hirsch and Donna Feldstein, in the same volume of the *Annals of the NY Academy* (vol. 437, 1984, p. 8-15), point out that "CMV mononucleosis often presents with prolonged fever, malaise, fatigue, anorexia (wasting syndrome?)." These symptoms are of course listed in various definitions of AIDS and pre-AIDS complex.

CMV can be isolated from the peripheral blood of both people with CMV-mononucleosis and people diagnosed with AIDS.

At least one report found that 98% of a group of African children tested positive for CMV antibodies. So the virus is apparently prevalent there.

JM Wallace in *Chest* (August 1987, vol. 2, p. 198-203) reviewed records and autopsy material of 54 patients who had been diagnosed with AIDS. 39 of these people had CMV infection documented by finding the virus in tissue samples. Of these, 23 had clearly been ill with a progressive form of CMV disease. In 2 patients who had had pneumonia, the only causative agent found was CMV (not pneumocystis).

MJ Post did a study of 10 AIDS patients who had central nervous system involvement. In autopsies, Post discovered CMV was implicated as an agent, and in 6 of these people CMV had caused an initial central nervous system infection which later instigated progressive encephalopathy and brought on death. (*AJR*, Jan. 1986, vol. 46, p. 1229-34)

In Harry Haverkos' study, "Factors Associated with the Pathogenesis of AIDS," (*Journal of Infectious Diseases*, vol. 156, July 1987), Haverkos indicates that "CMV is known to infect both T and B lymphocytes (immune-system elements). In addition, Giraldo et al have associated CMV with African KS (Kaposi's sarcoma)."

The above is a brief sampling of what's available on CMV in the medical literature. I cite these references, not to prove that CMV . causes anything, but only to imply that CMV could stand, in a fair fight, as good chance as HIV of being painted an agent of a thing called AIDS.

Its fate, however, is to remain in the background of merely opportunistic infections, second fiddle to HIV. When AIDS caught on as a singular idea of a single disease, when the clamps went in and the whole syndrome started to acquire notoriety, the obvious gambit was to press for novelty, a brand new virus. Congress was stirred to appropriate brand new money against a brand new threat.

So it was done.

No matter how much money is piled up on the doorstep of NIH, we need to sweep that building clean first, to put the money to work.

And even then, as far as alleviating-treatments are concerned, guerilla clinics, computer bulletin boards, doctors doing independent research, private research foundations, and the stories of AIDS survivors may all be more instructive than what cascades down from NIH.

IV DRUG USERS AND AIDS: A CONVERSATION WITH WILLIAM BURROUGHS

Real and obvious immunosuppression is put on the shelf and hidden by the obsessed attempt to prove that AIDS is one disease-entity caused by HIV.

In analyzing reported cases of AIDS among IV drug users, the fixation is on shared needles, as the route of HIV transmission. But what is the likelyhood that junkies would assist transmission of all sorts of microbes by sharing needles?

Novelist William Burroughs needs, as they say, no introduction. If the modern American novel has a forefront, Burroughs is there at the prow in his gray suit and fedora next to a stack of *Naked Lunch*, *Nova Express* and *Soft Machine*. He has written about and understands the world of the addict.

I spoke with him on March 19, 1988.

Q: Wasting away has now been incorporated into the symptom-list of AIDS. Haven't there always been some junkies who wasted away from using heroin?

A: That depends on how much they take. At three grains a day, they look like anybody. At an unreasonable seven grains, the change is remarkable. They have that wasted look. They make a rapid comeback, though. After they taper off the drug for a month, they look normal. I've seen (before and after) pictures of people in a facility in Hong Kong.

Q: They lose a lot of weight and gain it back?

A: That's right.

Q: Suppose they have a big habit and they aren't eating, or what they are eating has zero nutritive value, and they can't get into a treatment center. Then they could just keep wasting away.

A: Oh sure. In America, not many junkies can get themselves in that condition. They can't get enough junk.

They say junkies share needles, and that they can't afford to buy needles. If someone can get up fifty dollars a day for any sort of habit, he can pay two dollars for needles. For an outfit. Now the outfits, a plastic syringe and needle, are sold right in the drug drop for two dollars. There's no reason for them to share needles – unless some of them are ignorant beyond belief. They know about the danger of serum hepatitis. You can get serum hepatitis, malaria, and syphilis from sharing needles. Serum hepatitis is a very serious condition. So I wonder to what extent they are sharing needles. Have researchers gone out and interviewed all these people?

Q: I've seen one or two studies where they have.

A: Yes. I know there are cases where they do. I think this warrants a whole lot more study, though. This sexually transmitted disease (AIDS) has supposedly started in a population (IV drug users) that's notably asexual. A heavy heroin addict is almost completely non-sexual.

Q: So if you're not sharing needles and not having sex, where does the AIDS supposedly come from? You could cause some strange-looking illness with chemicals, especially when you're talking about contaminated drugs cut with who knows what.

A: Sure. It's such an unknown area when you don't know what the contaminants are. There was a case of poisoning they never analyzed that caused severe illness and blindness. The shipment was traced to Iran, then it hit Marseilles, Paris, and New York. I know someone who is virtually blind as a result of this stuff. It was an organic contaminant, but they never really pinned it down to exactly what. That was about six or seven years ago. They had a ward of these people in New York. About eight or ten.

. . . If they ever wanted to introduce a biologic or chemical agent, they'd have an ideal population in 250,000 addicts in New York. About 500,000 nationwide. By contamination at the source, namely the needles. Nothing would be simpler than to insert a tiny drop of blood into a needle and seal it up like a new needle. In fact, I've had people tell me they've bought needles, sealed up and found there was blood in the needles.

Q: And they've bought these needles from the person who sold them drugs?

A: Yes, exactly. Who in turn – someone comes to him and says, 'I've got ten thousand needles, good price.' The buyer is not going to examine them carefully. Nothing's easier than to contaminate a needle and then reseal it in a plastic container . . . It *could* have happened that way. That doesn't mean it *did*. One thing's for sure, if it was deliberate, they're not going to let it out.

Q: What about disposable versus old-style needles?

A: These disposable needles – you can't boil the syringe. It's made of plastic. I would venture to say almost all (junkies) are using disposables. The needles eventually get dull. You just keep changing the needles every week or so.

Q: Why share disposable needles if they're dirt cheap and plentiful?

A: I saw a columnist saying, 'They're so poor they have to share needles.' Well, that's absurd. The minimum to support a habit in New York would be thirty dollars a day. That'd just give you three shots. So most of them are running forty, fifty and sixty dollars a day. And up.

Q: I've heard that since the 1970s, there's a kind of ritual sharing of needles not related to economics.

A: I never heard of it. It seems to me it would be an idiotic ritual. Serum hepatitis is a hell of a thing. Very serious. And that is a way it's acquired, through contaminated needles.

Q: The drugs themselves are cut with something.

A: With anything.

Depending on severity, some symptoms of serum hepatitis include rash, weight loss, fatigue, loss of appetite, vomiting, cough and maliase. Once again, here is a non-AIDS condition that contains so-called AIDS and Pre-AIDS symptoms. Undoubtedly, junkies with hepatitis are being diagnosed as AIDS cases these days. The hysteria mandates it.   Since liver damage is such an ordinary fact among junkies, it wouldn't necessarily alert a doctor that hepatitis, not AIDS, was bringing about these symptoms.

CHAPTER THIRTY-ONE

THE POWER OF SUGGESTION AND THE AIDS BLOOD TEST

There is no way to measure the full effect of telling a person he has AIDS, or has tested positive for the "AIDS virus." These days, the distinction between a positive blood test and having AIDS is blurring over considerably. Doctors, unsure of themselves, are relying more and more, for diagnosis, on whether the patient is a member of a so-called high-risk group (male gay, IV drug user, sexual partner of a person who is gay or an IV drug user).

We have heard stories of people burning down the houses of those who tested positive for HIV. There has been suicide for the same reason.

In all of this, very few people have bothered to find out what it means to say a person:

a) is infected with the AIDS virus;

b) is an AIDS carrier;

c) is HIV-positive.

Hysteria is the guiding principle.

In fact, a), b), and c) all mean, in practical terms, the same thing. A person has registered positive on a blood test for HIV.

And, of course, very few people really bother to find out what *that* means.

That is unfortunate, since a major component of immunosuppression is the diagnosis itself, never mind what actual disease factors may or may not be present. Walking around with the belief that you are inhabited by a virus which is invariably fatal to you, day after day, can bring about some extremely debilitating effects. Particularly when estimates of date of death range from one to 16 years.

Of course, if the blood test is geared to HIV, which hasn't been proven to cause human disease, then the whole situation becomes quite crazy.

Naturally, with AIDS on people's minds, there is a great deal of pressure to make the blood test mandatory. Yet, researchers are in serious disagreement about which tests to use, how to use them.

If a wedge is going to be driven into society's fabric using this idea of a disease, if people are going to start polarizing groups in a serious way, by pitting one against another, testing is their mechanism

Let us assume, for purposes of discussion, that HIV is the cause of AIDS, in order to show that, even assuming an orthodox view of AIDS, mass testing is a hoax.

There are two exams which are normally called "AIDS tests" (although very expensive other procedures can be done, such as searching human tissue directly for the HIV virus). These two basic exams are the Elisa (also called EIA) and the Western blot.

The Elisa comes first. 5cc of blood are taken from the testee. What the lab then looks for are specific antibodies (part of the body's immune-defense forces) which have been generated against an intrusion of the HIV virus.

Antibodies are spread out on a plastic layer. If they are indeed antibodies specifically against the HIV virus, they will bind with viral proteins on the plastic. When this bound mixture is treated with chemicals, a color-change will occur, indicating a positive test.

Positive Elisas should then be validated by using the more specific "confirmatory," as it's called, Western blot test. Rather than a color-change, a recognizable pattern will emerge if HIV antibodies and viral proteins bind on a sheet of lab paper. The recognizable pattern equals a positive AIDS exam.

"Positive" is widely taken to mean: You have the AIDS virus in your body.

The FDA is the federal licensing agency for all U.S. AIDS testing. Their Washington office sent me a document simply titled *Summary and Explanation of the Test*, dated July 23, 1987 (and not on Agency letterhead):

"In order to afford maximum protection of the blood supply, the EIA (Elisa) test was designed to be extremely sensitive. As a result, non-specific (falsely positive) reactions may be seen in samples from some people . . . due to prior pregnancy, blood transfusions, or other exposure . . ."

In fact, other literature suggests that falsely positive Elisa tests can result from alcoholism, certain types of malignancies, autoimmune diseases, malaria, liver disease, heat-treating the blood sample to be tested, prolonged storage of plasma.

The FDA document recommends the following regimen: Have an Elisa. If it comes up positive, do *two* more Elisas. If either one of those additional Elisas turns up positive, do a confirmatory Western blot.

If the Western blot says positive, consider your entire test was positive. If the Western blot is negative, the overall results are uncertain.

If your first Elisa was positive, but neither of your next two Elisas were positive, consider you're negative.

"Negative" is widely taken to mean, you don't have the AIDS virus in your body.

So much for conventional wisdom. Now let's scratch below the surface.

From nearly the beginning of AIDS testing in the spring of 1985, health officials have raised questions as to its accuracy or meaning. In May of '85, the New Jersey State Public Health Council rejected a proposal to require all cases of positive AIDS tests in the state to be reported to health authorities. Dr. Robert Altman, chief of epidemiology for the State Health Department, cited part of the reason the proposal was turned down: "Exactly what a positive test result means is not that well defined at this point in time."

I asked the CDC's Gail Lloyd about such charges. She simply said, "Our scientists here consider the tests are pretty reliable."

But, for example, there are clearly problems proving an AIDS test is negative. This past spring, physicians Christopher Damm and Louis Aledort, of the Mount Sinai School of Medicine in New York, responded in the *New York Times* to an organization which claimed

267

it was "the first dating service in New York requiring members to prove they are not infected with the AIDS virus."

Damm and Aledort said: "Given the status of (AIDS) antibody testing, we believe that this claim ('romance without risk') is inaccurate.

"Antibody testing usually produces positive results 30 days to six months after initial exposure to the virus. The period between exposure and a positive blood test is called a 'window.' During this time a person can transmit the virus even though his or her blood test is negative.

"Given the reasonable chance of transmission during the window period, we would suggest that individuals approach any new sexual partner who has tested negative with the same caution as one would approach a partner who has not been tested."

Not very comforting. But since this *New York Times* comment, the window may have gotten disconcertingly bigger. A recent study in the British medical journal *Lancet* by Dr. Kai Krohn reveals that in one group of men, 15% had repeated negative AIDS tests and yet were otherwise found to have had the virus dating back *10-34 months*.

If you meticulously followed the implications of this new study, you would get tested every few months for three years after sex with a new partner – in the meantime abstaining from sex with anyone else – just to make sure you weren't passing on the virus.

The bottom line? A negative AIDS blood test could mean you're negative for the virus, or it could mean the test isn't registering that you're actually positive yet.

On the phone, Dr. J.D. Robinson, who reported on the *Lancet* study in the *Wall Street Journal*, emphasized the value of AIDS testing in a clinical setting "where you have a patient who has symptoms. Testing then can be a useful tool . . . also when combined with other blood indicators. This is quite different from thinking about 500,000 statistical tests done on a mass screening basis."

Robinson indicated that new more accurate AIDS tests, which may eventually be used in mass-screening programs, are in various stages of development.[1]

A UCLA virologist bluntly told me there are unknown factors in AIDS tests.

Q: A positive Elisa test means the person . . .

A: . . . has been exposed to the AIDS virus.

Q: Can we guarantee whether the virus is now in his body or isn't in his body?

A: We don't know that.

Q: Do we know who, coming up with a positive AIDS test, is infectious to others, or under what conditions he could become infectious?

A: No.

The virologist then added, "It's (sometimes) possible that a positive AIDS test is positive for another virus (not HIV)."

A few days after this conversation, I encountered a physician who took personal offense at my investigation of AIDS testing. 1) He refused to go on the record, and 2) he said, "The furor in the press over this testing thing is ridiculous. You people are trying to decide important matters over the telephone. These questions belong in reputable medical journals."

In other words, a reporter's job is merely to relay science-news direct from the press people at the CDC to the public, untainted by thought.

I decided I would peruse a few venerable medical journals and see what professionals in the field had to say about AIDS testing. Of course, esteemed researchers would all maintain that testing was efficient, worthwhile and deeply meaningful. Certainly. After all, wasn't that what the press was telling us? Weren't the politicians echoing it too? They had to be getting their info from the highest medical authorities.

---

[1] The pharmaceutical house, Smith, Kline, has recently announced a new test. It claims it is far more accurate than current tests.

Anon, forthwith, and hence are the results of letting my fingers do the walking through medical journals of the last several years. As you'll immediately see, what the popular press and the scientific bureaucrats tell the public about AIDS testing is one thing; what the researchers report in their journals is quite, quite another thing.

Let's start with the March 1987 issue of the *Journal of Clinical Microbiology*. James Carlson, of the University of California at Davis' School of Pathology, drops this bombshell. He says that in low-risk groups, the false-positive rate in Elisa tests is an overwhelming "84.2% in our study and 77.1% recently reported by the American Red Cross . . ."

N.B: A false-positive AIDS test means you appear to have AIDS-virus antibodies, *but you really don't.*

Carlson continues: "It must be noted that even though we feel the Western blot technique is presently the most acceptable method...Western blot analysis is a subjective method with quality control limitations; the possibility of false-positive results still exists. Therefore, we hope that new, more specific objective approaches will soon be available to provide definitive results for HIV serology."

Next, I picked up a copy of the January 9, 1986 *New England Journal of Medicine*. Dr. Michael Saag of the University of Alabama and Judith Britz, Ph.D., of Electro-Nucleonics, Inc. reported on the case of a 34-year-old woman from rural Alabama. She'd donated blood and was routinely tested for AIDS. Her Elisa came up positive. She had no AIDS symptoms. She was married and monogamous. Her other blood studies were normal.

So four more Elisa tests were done on her. They all showed positive, too. One backup Western blot was done. It showed strongly positive. How certain can you get?

Then new blood was drawn from her and sent around to a handful of prestigious labs for retesting. Now all Elisa and Western blots were *negative*.

Then the Elisas were repeated at two of these labs. They were both *positive*.

"Western blot tests," the authors conclude, ". . . have been used as the 'gold standard' by which other tests (e.g. the Elisa) are judged to be falsely positive . . . the need for improved confirmatory tests . . . is evident."

Dr. Saag and Ms. Britz point out that a number of factors will cause false-positives on Elisa tests: antibodies to nuclear antigens, human leukocyte antigens and human T-cells antigens. Apparently, the Alabama lady had antibodies to mitochondria. They'd wreaked havoc with her test results.

In the December 1986 *American Journal of Medicine*, Dr. Rahmat Afrasiabi reports on just the opposite sort of occurrence. Three male homosexual AIDS patients with Kaposi's sarcoma turned out not to have any antibodies to the HIV virus at all. In other words, their AIDS tests were negative.

Between May of 1983 and June of 1985, blood samples were collected from these men. Using two different Elisa test kits and the Western blot, "testing of serum from these patients (was) negative for (HIV) antibodies," Afrasiabi reports.

Have you been reading about such findings in your local papers?

British researcher L.J. Oldham, writing in the *Journal of Medical Virology* (January 1987), concludes after running tests of blood which was weakly positive for HIV antibodies, "Our findings suggest that Western blot cannot be depended upon as the sole confirmatory test for (HIV)."

Later in the same paper, Oldham states: "As has been shown, Western blot . . . lacks full sensitivity and specificity."

And finally: ". . . confirmatory procedures are at present beyond the scope of most screening laboratories."

There is more.

Evelyn Lennette, in the February 1987 *Journal of Clinical Microbiology*, indicates that "both of these assays (Elisa and Western blot) have drawbacks . . . (there are) reports of both false-positive and false-negative results with the Elisa, necessitating the use of a second confirmatory test . . . The immunoblot (Western blot) is also not free from false results."

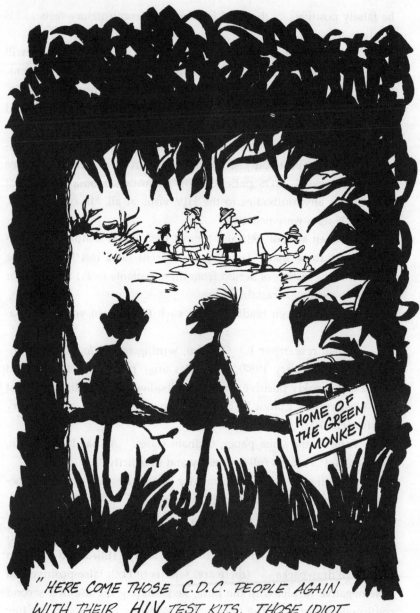

"HERE COME THOSE C.D.C. PEOPLE AGAIN WITH THEIR HIV TEST KITS. THOSE IDIOT HUMANS'LL DO ANYTHING FOR GRANT MONEY!"

Lennette and her co-authors suggest using a different confirmatory test, the IFA procedure. But, in other journal literature, the IFA has been compared unfavorably with the Elisa-Western blot one-two sequence.

On top of these journal statements, several sources indicated to me that from testing-lab to lab, results may vary according to technicians – particularly with the Western blot. How does a layperson choose a "good" testing lab? No one I spoke with could answer that other than by saying, "Find a doctor whose judgment you trust."

An interesting ploy some researchers attempt in defending testing is the invocation of risk-groups (such as gay males and IV drug users). In the September 15, 1986, issue of *Post Graduate Medicine*, a magazine sent out to educate primary-care physicians, Dr. Francis D. Pien asserts: "The predictive value of a positive (Elisa) result *depends on the incidence of (HIV) disease in the population group represented.*" (emphasis added) Pien then says that in certain high-risk groups, "the incidence of (HIV) antibodies approaches 70%."

Translation: If you're already very probably carrying the AIDS virus, the unreliability of the tests will be offset by the fact that you're probably positive. This approaches nonsense.

In fact, in the FDA document, *Summary and Explanation of the Test* which was sent to me, there is a cautionary note on just this subject: "Although . . . both the degree of risk for HIV infection . . . and the degree of reactivity of the serum (test results) may be of value in interpreting the test, these correlations are imperfect."

Let me stack a few more logs on the pyre. In the July-August 1985 issue of the journal *Transfusion.*, Paul Holland considers the case of 1280 blood donors whose blood was tested by the Elisa test kits of two different manufacturers. The Abbott Elisa located 20 positive tests on first reading. On repeat-examination, 5 stayed positive. Then the Elisa of a company called ENI was used on this same group of 1280 specimens. The ENI Elisa kit found 25 samples positive on first reading. On retest, 14 samples stayed positive.

And only three donors, as it turned out, were positive on both Elisa kits from both companies. Finally . . . *none* of the Elisas were confirmed positive by a Western blot.

In some ways, the most disturbing analysis of both the Elisa and the Western blot tests comes from Dr. Harvey Fineberg, Dean of the Harvard School of Public Health. Fineberg published a statistical study on AIDS testing in the spring of 1987, in *Law, Medicine and Health Care.*

"To begin with," Fineberg told me on the phone, "in the study, we accepted the advertised accuracy ratings of the Elisa test. It's reportedly able to find true positives at a rate of 93.4%, and it supposedly can detect true negatives correctly 99.78% of the time.

"So let's say that 3 out of 10,000 people in the U.S. are really infected with the HIV virus. If we consider a sample of 100,000 people, that means 30 will actually be infected with HIV. The Elisa test will be able to pinpoint 93.4%, or 28 of those people.

"On the other side of the ledger, that leaves 99,970 out of 100,000 who are truly *not* infected with the AIDS virus.

"If the Elisa is 99.78% capable of finding these real negatives, it will locate 99,750 of these people without fail. That leaves 220 negatives it missed (the difference between 99,970 and 99,750). How did it miss? By calling those 220 people *positive* when they weren't.

"So now you have, out of every 100,000 people, 28 truly positive and 220 falsely positive test results. That means the statistical chances are about 90% that a positive-reading Elisa is wrongly positive."

Fineberg continued: "A second Elisa won't change that either. If you do a Western blot, the odds might, at best, be lowered to 25%. In other words, a fourth of the time, a positive AIDS test would be falsely positive."

A test that's wrong 25% of the time. Not very comforting odds.

"If I had a patient who was really engaging in high-risk behavior," Fineberg said, "I wouldn't rely on test results. I'd simply sit down with this person and try to make him see he needed to change his lifestyle."

Michael Marmor, associate professor at NYU's Medical Center, partially agrees with Dr. Fineberg. In a letter to the *New York Times* (May 16, 1987), Marmor states that only 36% of those in low-risk groups who test positive on an Elisa "would be infected (with HIV). A positive result, thus, could not be given much credence."

However, Marmor then goes on to say that using the Western blot as a backup, "almost all false-positive results are eliminated while true-positives are retained."

He is obviously at odds with some of the researchers whose critical remarks about the Western blot I've quoted here. Such fundamental disagreement in the professional ranks is not a recommendation for taking AIDS testing seriously. Or to put it another way, government promotion of AIDS testing as nearly flawless is scandalous.

At this point, I was faced with odd prospects. I queried several physicians about what I'd dug up in the medical literature. They weren't familiar with the above studies, with the heavy criticism of the Western blot, or with Harvey Fineberg's article.

About all I got from these doctors was, "I haven't seen the articles you're referring to. As far as I know, the AIDS tests are reliable." An apparent case of physicians not reading their own literature.

I then spoke with Peter Drotman, an internationally known epidemiologist at the CDC. Drotman began by saying that both the Elisa and Western blot are "extraordinarily good techniques for detecting antibodies."

Then, in direct contradiction to the FDA stance (as well as that of many other researchers), Drotman said: "The Western blot is not a confirmatory test. The Elisa and the Western blot are two different tests both used to detect antibodies."

Drotman indicated, "We'd like to have a real confirmatory test."

I then pointed out one of the criticisms of the Western blot: that it needs to be more standardized to qualify for clinical use. "Yes," Drotman said, "the Western blot should be more standardized . . . there is variance, depending on the lab doing it. But, if it's well done, it's a good test."

275

Again, the obvious question for the consumer who's thinking of getting AIDS tested is, how do you know you've found a good lab?

I found Drotman's remark about the Western blot not being a confirmatory test pretty explosive. There are many physicians and researchers who concede that the Elisa is frought with problems – but when validated or directly contradicted by a Western blot, they feel the status of the testee then becomes clear. Taken with the criticism of the Western blot in the medical literature I'd found, Drotman's position seemed to throw the whole reliability of testing *further* into question.

Next, I spoke with another quite well-known researcher at the CDC, Harold Jaffe. He also readily admitted that "there is a problem with a confirmatory test for AIDS . . . (Western blot) is a difficult test. There is only one real type of kit, although some labs have developed their own. Nobody is all that happy with the Western blot . . . In a high-risk person, chances are that if both tests (Elisa and Western blot) are positive, the person is positive."

I then asked Jaffe about Holland's 1985 *Transfusion* study, which showed such variance between Elisa kits manufactured by different companies.

"There is some variance among commercial (Elisa) kits licensed in the U.S.," he said. "It's not as much a problem as it was when testing first started, back in 1985 . . . but there is still some variance."

"The overall point," Jaffe concluded, "is that the tests are quite good – as good as other tests."

Q: It seems there is a problem with AIDS testing – a doctor is most often dealing with people who have no symptoms. In other tests, you have the patient in your office and he has a disease you can diagnose. Then, with a test on top of *that* . . .

A: Yes . . . it's foolish to tell low-risk people they're infected on one test. If I – and I consider myself low-risk – came up positive, I'd ask my doctor to draw another blood sample.

Q: Start all over again.

A: Yes. Do a new series of tests. If a person just wants to get tested because he's curious – he's low-risk – he slept with a prostitute three years ago and it's nagging him – then okay, but don't take a positive test as absolute. Run through the tests again with another blood sample."

This high-risk group, low-risk group business seemed to inflect everyone's conversation about the reliability of AIDS-testing. If you were a white male heterosexual, for example, you were part of a group among which there were only 220 diagnosed cases of full-blown AIDS in the U.S. Therefore, according to this loose doctrine, if faced with a positive Elisa and Western blot, you would ask for a fresh round of tests. On the other hand, if you were a male homosexual, you should possibly accept the first run of tests as gospel if the reading was positive.

Yet, as the FDA stated, there was no conclusive correlation, certainly no numerical formula, for combining and meshing your risk-factor for HIV with the test results. No, this was a vague gray area. Both Elisa and the Western blot were very prone to error based on factors in no way connected to one's risk of developing AIDS or antibodies to HIV.

Finally, I talked with another high-ranking epidemiologist at the National Institutes of Health. Owing to a misunderstanding, he thought he was just filling in background for me off the record. I decided to let his comments stand and omit his name.

I pointed out the apparent lack of a numerical formula to combine risk-factor and test-reliability.

"Yes," he said, "that's a principle of testing in general . . . (with AIDS tests) you *could* make formula-predictions (if) you knew the odds (for carrying AIDS antibodies) of the high-risk group *as a number* . . . (but) we don't have that figure.

In fact, I feel one of the groups at highest risk for AIDS, male white homosexuals . . . things are changing there (getting better) because they've changed their (sexual) behavior . . . so that makes it even harder to predict (risk as a number)."

At this point, 3 things seemed apparent to me:

1) Researchers had reported serious accuracy-problems with both types of AIDS tests.

2) Other researchers maintained the tests were excellent, so there were very unresolved differences of opinion.

3) Attempts to make the tests seem more accurate by invoking risk-groups were going to be of marginal help to people getting tests.

AIDS testing has *serious* problems.

Begin with a test for antibodies to a virus. The test is promoted as a means to isolate so-called infectious carriers. The test is flawed badly, both in a statistical sense and from the point of view of lab science. Nevertheless, the test is pushed and foisted on the public, and sold hard to legislators who may begin to believe their constituencies deep down want this mandatory exam to be performed.

Meanwhile, the press cooperates by broadcasting quotes about the test which assume it is a reliable tool.

As hysteria is headlined, as predictions mount about the millions of deaths just over the horizon, more people enlist into the camp of those who are absolutely sure AIDS is one entity caused invariably and only by HIV. Grant monies believe it, too, and scientists who are worried about their car and house payments forget their doubts and join up on the side of HIV – they apply for grants under the aegis of supporting scientific truth.

As the disease's definition broadens, numbers of cases of AIDS swell;[2] even people who know there is a definitional shuffle-hustle accept that AIDS is on the increase in a big way. Pure hypnotism.

Though prominent figures like Harvey Fineberg, Dean of the Harvard School of Public Health, warn us about the intrinsic flaws concerning mass AIDS blood-testing, this kind of sensible information is buried under a tide of fear, under a demand for *more* testing.

At this point, elements of our society usually lumped together as "radical right" begin to see glimmers of their dreams coming true: the election of more strong leaders who are sure all the permissive living of the last two decades is coming home to roost. These leaders, of course, want to give this country back primacy of the authoritarian family, celibacy before marriage – except for the really top-drawer

---

[2] A recent study indicates that, since the 1987 CDC definition of AIDS has been disseminated, AIDS cases from San Francisco have increased by 19%, purely on the basis of this expanded definition. *JAMA*, Apr. 15, 1988, p. 2235.

people who can crawl around on all fours in expensive hotel rooms with strange outfits on and offer employment to prostitutes in our free capitalist society.

With the advent of a virus which can tie together a half-starving African trying to scratch out a meal from a bit of dry ground, and a gay male San Franciscan who is trying to get yet one more script filled for tetracycline, and the junky looking for a little envelope, and the indigent Haitian, and the French businessman who just came back from Zaire . . . can new prescription drugs and vaccines be far behind?

The discovery of a new germ brings Nobels as it brings profits to testing companies as it brings a new chance to separate the clean from the unclean, the righteous from the evil.

A momentum increases on all fronts, people in diverse sectors of the society begin to see a community of interest emerge. It begins to penetrate the minds of some people that they are riding on the same boat, and that the boat is a reliable vessel, it brings reward.

For those who feel that we are dealing with a disease that comes straight from God with a message attached to it, the disease is tolerable, since the AIDS scarlet sign is being pinned to people of the darker races, to homosexuals, to drug users and to the apparently promiscuous. If the drugs used to treat these people have unfortunate side-effects, that is tolerable too.

EPILOGUE

This is the chapter for several leftover thoughts, things I couldn't squeeze into other chapters, conclusions after looking back over the landscape.

First, a couple of replies to familiar arguments. As I mentioned earlier, devotees of HIV tend to warn that if you say HIV isn't causing disease, this will encourage people to go out and become promiscuous. The reply to that is, incidents of STDs (and attendant antibiotic-dosing) add up to lots of immunosuppression on their own. So one doesn't need HIV-terrorism to induce people to consider safer sex.

Second, the HIV-mob likes to point out that drugs and chemicals have been used for decades without causing AIDS; and there are countries now where dangerous chemicals are sold and yet those countries have no AIDS. Well, as I've said ten or twelve times in this book, the pattern of AIDS is: immune-suppression plus opportunistic infections. That pattern, under any name, has existed forever and in all countries. So whether a farm worker in Guatemala who is wasting away from exposure to a pesticide is *said* to have AIDS means nothing. He has terribly reduced immune-response, and he is developing infections.

There is a cute attitude, of course, among HIV researchers that the brand of immunosuppression they are uncovering is unique. If anything, I'm afraid, has been proven by their work over the last seven years, it is that they are *speculating* on the brand of immuno-suppression HIV is supposed to be causing. Destroyed T-cells, ruined macrophages, etc. These disease processes are mirrored, anyway, by the indistinguishable work of malnutrition, for example. Besides which, immune-response is a much broader activity than what the T-cells do.

So-called pediatric AIDS has become a major focus of late. Like transfusion-AIDS, it is a very emotional way of "proving" how devastating AIDS is. But infant death in the US has been on the rise for various reasons; in the following appendix, there is a reference to the DPT vaccination as a hidden cause of sudden infant death. Babies are very vulnerable to infection, because their immunity is not yet established. When they receive transfusions, the door opens to multiple infections by many germs. Under the rubric of an HIV-positive blood test, it is very easy to say that *whatever* a baby is suffering from, it is AIDS.

When the people who were sent out to track AIDS, in the first place, left their offices, their heads were full of HIV-dogma and survey-type questions to ask gay men and IV drug users. They ventured into neighborhoods, they set up shop at universities and did extensive interviews. But one thing that never really occurred to them to do was: Get people who have been on the scene to *describe* what had been happening in their world. Get stories. Get real leads and then follow them up. Discover the contaminated drugs. Figure out what had been happening to people's health at ground-level. There are lots of smart folks out there who know a hell of a lot more about, say, gay life than epidemiologists coming in from uptown labs.

So much has been not discovered because of the antiseptic personality of this sort of survey resarch.

For example, here is yet another footnote on drugs on the gay scene. PharmChem Labs of Menlo Park, California, reports that strychnine, the lethal poison, was an occasional adulterant of amphetamines and MDA in the 1970s. It was added to these street drugs apparently as a stimulant, in very small amounts. Some people died from it. The effects of taking strychnine-laced speed over a long period of time would be, needless to say, very deleterious. It would suppress a number of immune responses in the body. Of course, without knowing this poison was on the scene, no doctor would check for it in his weakening patients.

Yes, speed wasn't just used in the gay communities of San Francisco, New York, and LA, but it was used there in very large quantities; and speed burnouts are a kind of wasting-away, regardless of who the victim is. In the hetero community, the diagnosis isn't AIDS, because a medical reflex-action hasn't developed, in which AIDS symptoms in heterosexuals are immediately tabbed as AIDS-like; whereas in homosexuals anything remotely resembling AIDS is often sufficient for a diagnosis.

The story of strychnine, however, doesn't become part of the body of knowledge about AIDS. No, the researchers who get out into the street have their survey-forms ready; they are headed in a different direction. They don't, for example, hear about people in LA on the gay scene dying after long and heavy use of crystal meth, their immunity shot. They don't hear now about some gay men who think that wearing condoms is the only thing they need to do to protect themselves, that tons of crystal meth are okay.

After such a failure as AIDS-research, in all its aspects, the most intelligent thing to do for the health of the US may be to cut off funding for NIH, disband it, dismantle the buildings, throw some seed on the ground, forget it was ever there and start over. Start over with the premise that health is supposed to benefit people. It has nothing necessarily to do with selling cascades of new pharmaceuticals. It doesn't have anything to do with winning Laskers and Nobels. If a researcher likes shucking the public, let him go into selling. If he enjoys participating in useless and false research in a silent way, let him become a speechwriter. But get him out of public health.

Start over. Say, "Boys, we're not committed to anything but better health. That's all. No axes to grind. Anything goes, as long as it works and as long as side effects are REALLY negligible. No flag-waving. No viral heroics. No posturing. No baloney. Research any damn things you want to. As many as you can. Just improve health."

Imagine how much would have to change to effect this sort of revolution. Then you know why health is the biggest consumer movement in America.

APPENDICES
1-7

APPENDIX 1

VACCINES AS IMMUNOSUPPRESSION

For years, critics on the fringes of medicine have pointed to problems with vaccines. It is generally acknowledged that, given to people whose immune systems are compromised, they can be immunosuppressive.[1]   And from time to time, stories have surfaced about vaccines which have been contaminated by extraneous viruses or bacteria, as a result of the manufacturing process.

We are taught to believe that untoward reactions to vaccines are rare, and that there has never been a question about the overwhelming success of all vaccines at all times, wherever they have been used.

The recent history of vaccines, though, shows a much more spotty record than one might think. In fact, it raises very disturbing questions about what vaccines do and don't do to the human body. Here is simply a series of excerpts from several authors on the subject. It is a quite different slant on vaccines.

"The combined death rate from scarlet fever, diphtheria, whooping cough and measles among children up to fifteen shows that nearly 90 percent of the total decline in mortality between 1860 and 1965 had occurred before the introduction of antibiotics and widespread immunization. In part, this recession may be attributed to improved housing and to a decrease in the virulence of micro-organisms, but by far the most important factor was a higher host-resistance due to better nutrition."

---

[1] This is particularly true in the Third World, where large numbers of people suffer from malnutrition. It can also be true among people whose immune-response has been dampened by drugs.

Ivan Illich, *Medical Nemesis* (Bantam Books, 1977)

"The principal evidence that . . . vaccines are effective actually dates from the more recent period, during which time the dreaded polio epidemics of the 1940s and 1950s have never reappeared in the developed countries; and measles, mumps and rubella, which even a generation ago were among the commonest diseases of childhood, have become far less prevalent, at least in their classic acute forms, since the triple MMR vaccine was introduced into common use.

"Yet how the vaccines actually accomplish these changes is not nearly as well understood as most people like to think it is. The disturbing possibility they they act in some other way than by producing a genuine immunity is suggested by the fact that the diseases in question have continued to break out even in highly immunized populations, and that in such cases the observed differences in incidence and severity between immunized and unimmunized persons have tended to be far less dramatic than expected, and in some cases, not measurably significant at all.

"In a recent British outbreak of whooping cough, for example, even fully immunized children contracted the disease in fairly large numbers; and the rates of serious complications and death were reduced only slightly (5). In another recent outbreak of pertussis, 46 of the 85 fully immunized children studied eventually contracted the disease (6).

"In 1977, 34 new cases of measles were reported on the campus of UCLA, in a population that was supposedly 91% immune, according to careful serological testing (7). Another 20 cases of measles were reported in the Pecos, New Mexico, area within a period of a few months in 1981, and 75% of them had been fully immunized, some of them quite recently (8). A survey of sixth-graders in a well-immunized urban community revealed that about 15% of this age group are still susceptible to rubella, a figure essentially identical with that of the pre-vaccine era (9).

"Finally, although the overall incidence of typical acute measles in the U.S. has dropped sharply from about 400,000 cases annually in the early 1960s to about 30,000 cases by 1974-76, the death rate remained exactly the same (10); and, with the peak incidence now occurring in adolescents and young adults, the risk of pneumonia and demonstrable liver abnormalities has actually increased substantially, according to one recent study, to well over 3% and 2%, respectively (11)."

Richard Moskowitz, MD, *The Case Against Immunizations*, 1983, American Institute of Homeopathy.

(5) Stewart, G., "Vaccination Against Whooping Cough: Efficiency vs. Risks," *Lancet*, 1977, p. 234.

(6) *Medical Tribune*, Jan. 10, 1979, p. 1.

(7) Cherry, J., "The New Epidemiology of Measles and Rubella," *Hospital Practice*, July 1980, pp. 52-54.

(8) Unpublished data from the New Mexico Health Department (private communication).

(9) Lawless, M., et al, "Rubella Susceptibility in Sixth-Graders," *Pediatrics* 65: 1086-1089, June, 1980.

(10) Cherry, *op. cit.*, p. 49.

(11) *Infectious Diseases*, January, 1982, p. 21.

"Of all reported whooping cough cases between 1979 and 1984 in children over 7 months of age – that is, old enough to have received the primary course of the DPT shots (diphtheria, pertussis, tetanus) – 41% occurred in children who had received three or more shots and 22% in children who had one or two immunizations.

"Among children under 7 months of age who had whooping cough, 34% had been immunized between one and three times . . .

". . . Based on the only U.S. findings on adverse DPT reactions, an FDA-financed study at the University of California, Los Angeles, one out of every 350 children will have a convulsion; one in 180 children will experience high-pitched screaming; and one in 66 will have a fever of 105 degrees or more."[2]

Jennifer Hyman, *Democrat and Chronicle*, Rochester, New York, special supplement on DPT, dated April, 1987.

---

2 All of these reactions are indicative of possible brain-damage.

"A study undertaken in 1979 at the University of California, Los Angeles, under the sponsorship of the Food and Drug Administration, and which has been confirmed by other studies, indicates that in the U.S.A. approximately 1,000 infants die annually as a direct result of DPT vaccinations, and these are classified as SIDS (Sudden Infant Death Syndrome) deaths. These represent about 10 to 15% of the total number of SIDS deaths occurring annually in the U.S.A. (between 8,000 and 10,000 depending on which statistics are used)."

Leon Chaitow, *Vaccination and Immunization*, CW Daniel Company Limited, Saffron Walden, Essex, England, 1987.

"Assistant Secretary of Health Edward Brandt, Jr., MD, testifying before the U.S. Senate Committee on Labor and Human Resources, rounded . . . figures off to 9,000 cases of convulsions, 9,000 cases of collapse, and 17,000 cases of high-pitched screaming for a total of 35,000 acute neurological reactions occurring within forty-eight hours of a DPT shot among America's children every year."

DPT: A Shot in the Dark, by Harris L. Coulter and Barbara Loe Fischer, Harcourt Brace Jovanovich.

"While 70-80% of British children were immunized against pertussis in 1970-71, the rate is now 39%. The committee predicts that the next pertussis epidemic will probably turn out to be more severe than the one in 1974/75. However, they do not explain why, in 1970/71, there were more than 33,000 cases of pertussis with 41 fatal cases among the very well immunized British child population; whereas in 1974/75, with a declining rate of vaccination, a pertussis epidemic caused only 25,000 cases with 25 fatalities."

Wolfgang Ehrengut, *Lancet*, Feb. 18, 1978, p. 370.

". . . Barker and Pichichero, in a prospective study of 1232 children in Denver, Colorado, found after DTP that only 7% of those vaccinated were free from untoward reactions, which included pyrexia (53%), acute behavioral changes (82%), prolonged screaming (13%), and listlessness, anorexia and vomiting. 71% of those receiving second injections of DTP experienced two or more of the reactions monitored."

Lancet, May 28, 1983, p. 1217

"Publications by the World Health Organization show that diphtheria is steadily declining in most European countries, including those in which there has been no immunization. The decline began long before vaccination was developed. There is certainly no guarantee that vaccination will protect a child against the disease; in fact, over 30,000 cases of diphtheria have been recorded in the United Kingdom in fully immunized children."

Leon Chaitow, *Vaccination and Immunization*, p. 58.

"Pertussis (whooping cough) immunization is controversial, as the side effects have received a great deal of publicity. The counter claim is that the effectiveness and protection offered by the procedure far outweigh the possible ill effects . . . annual deaths, per million children, from this disease over the period from 1900 to the mid-nineteen seventies, shows that from a high point of just under 900 deaths per million children (under age 15) in 1905, the decline has been consistent and dramatic. There had been a lowering of mortality rates of approximately 80% by the time immunization was introduced on a mass scale, in the mid-nineteen fifties. The decline has continued, albeit at a slower rate, ever since. No credit can be given to vaccination for the major part of the decline since it was not in use."

Chaitow, *Vaccination and Immunization*, p. 63.

". . . the swine-flu vaccination program was one of its (CDC) greatest blunders.

"It all began in 1976 when CDC scientists saw that a virus involved in a flu attack outbreak at Fort Dix, N.J., was similar to the swine-flu virus that killed 500,000 Americans in 1918. Health officials immediately launched a 100-million dollar program to immunize every American. But the expected epidemic never materialized, and the vaccine led to partial paralysis in 532 people. There were 32 deaths."

U.S. News and World Report, Joseph Carey, October 14, 1985, p. 70, "How Medical Sleuths Track Killer Diseases."

"Despite (cases) in which (smallpox) vaccination plainly failed to protect the population, and despite the rampant side-effects of the methods, the proponents of vaccination continued their attempts to justify the methods by claims that the disease had declined in Europe as a whole during the period of its compulsory use. If the decline could be correlated with the use of the vaccination, then all else could be set aside, and the advantage between its current low incidence could be shown to outweigh the periodic failures of the method, and to favour the continued use of vaccination. However, the credit for the decline in the incidence of smallpox could not be given to vaccination. The fact is that its incidence declined in all parts of Europe, whether or not vaccination was employed."

Chaitow, *Vaccination and Immunization,* pp. 6-7.

"Smallpox, like typhus, has been dying out (in England) since 1780. Vaccination in this country has largely fallen into disuse since people began to realize how its value was discredited by the great smallpox epidemic of 1871-2 (which occurred after extensive vaccination)."[3]

W. Scott Webb, *A Century of Vaccination,* Swan Sonnenschein, 1898.

On May 8, 1985, 155 member states unanimously accepted the finding of the WHO Global Commission for the Certification of Smallpox Eradication:

1. "Smallpox eradication has been achieved throughout the world.

2. "There is no evidence that smallpox will return as an epidemic disease."

---

[3] Another English physician, Dr. Charles Creighton, reported that in 1871, in Bavaria there were 30,742 cases of smallpox, of which 29,429 had been previously vaccinated.

"In this incident (Kyoto, Japan, 1948) – the most serious of its kind – a toxic batch of alum-precipitated toxoid (APT) was responsible for illness in over 600 infants and for no fewer than 68 deaths.

"On 20 and 22 October, 1948, a large number of babies and children in the city of Kyoto received their first injection of APT. On the 4th and 5th of November, 15,561 babies and children aged some months to 13 years received their second dose. One to two days later, 606 of those who had been injected fell ill. Of these, 9 died of acute diphtheritic paralysis in seven to fourteen days, and 59 of late paralysis mainly in four to seven weeks."

Sir Graham Wilson, *Hazards of Immunization*, Athone Press, University of London, 1967.

"Accidents may, however, follow the use of this so-called killed (rabies) vaccine owing to inadequate processing. A very serious occurrence of this sort occurred at Fortaleza, Ceara, Brazil, in 1960. No fewer than 18 out of 66 persons vaccinated with Fermi's carbolized (rabies) vaccine suffered from encephalomyelitis and every one of the eighteen died."

Sir Graham Wilson, *Hazards of Immunization*.

"At a press conference in Washington on 24 July, 1942, the Secretary of War reported that 28,585 cases of jaundice had been observed in the (American) Army between 1 January and 4 July after yellow fever vaccination, and of these 62 proved fatal."

Wilson, *Hazards of Immunization*.

"The world's biggest trial (conducted in south India) to assess the value of BCG tuberculosis vaccine has made the startling revelation that the vaccine 'does not give any protection against bacillary forms of tuberculosis.' The study said to be 'most exhaustive and meticulous,' was launched in 1968 by the Indian Council of Medical Research (ICMR) with assistance from the World Health Organization (WHO) and the U.S. Centers for Disease Control in Atlanta, Georgia."

"The incidence of new cases among the BCG vaccinated group was slightly (but statistically insignificantly) higher than in the control group, a finding that led to the conclusion that BCG's protective effect 'was zero.'"

New Scientist, November 15, 1979, as quoted by Hans Ruesch in *Naked Empress,* Civis Publishers, Switzerland, 1982.

"Between 10 December 1929 and 30 April 1930, 251 of 412 infants born in Lubeck received three doses of BCG vaccine by the mouth during the first ten days of life. Of these 251, 72 died of tuberculosis, most of them in two to five months and all but one before the end of the first year. In addition, 135 suffered from clinical tuberculosis but eventually recovered; and 44 became tuberculin-positive but remained well. None of the 161 unvaccinated infants born at the time was affected in this way and none of these died of tuberculosis within the following three years."

Hazards of Immunization, Wilson.

"We conducted a randomized double-blind placebo-controlled trial to test the efficacy of the 14-valent pneumococcal capsular polysaccharide vaccine in 2295 high-risk patients . . . Seventy-one episodes of proved or probable pneumococcal pneumonia or bronchitis occurred among 63 of the patients (27 placebo recipients and 36 vaccine recipients) . . . We were unable to demonstrate any efficacy of the pneumococcal vaccine in preventing pneumonia or bronchitis in this population."

New England Journal of Medicine, November 20, 1986, p. 1318, Michael Simberkoff et al.

In the spring of 1955, Cutter Labs started selling their standard polio vaccine. The vaccine was infective, and 200 cases of polio resulted among vaccinees. Of these, there were eleven deaths. About 100 cases of paralysis resulted. JR

"But already before Salk developed his vaccine, polio had been constantly regressing; the 39 cases out of every 100,000 inhabitants registered in 1942 had gradually diminished from year to year until they were reduced to only 15 cases in 1952. . . according to M. Beddow Baylay, the English surgeon and medical historian."

Slaughter of the Innocent, Hans Reusch, Civitas Publishers, Switzerland, and Swain, New York, 1983.

"Many published stories and reports have stated, implied and otherwise led professional people and the public to believe that the sharp reduction of cases (and of deaths) from poliomyelitis in 1955 as compared to 1954 is attributable to the Salk vaccine . . . That it is a misconception follows from these considerations. The number of children inoculated has been too small to account for the decrease. The sharp decrease was apparent before the inoculations began or could take effect and was of the same order as the decrease following the immediate post-inoculation period."

Dr. Herbert Ratner, *Child and Family*, vol. 20, no. 1, 1987.

"So far it is hardly possible to gain insight into the extent of the immunization catastrophe of 1955 in the United States. It may be considered certain that the officially ascertained 200 cases which were caused directly or indirectly by the (polio) vaccination constitute minimum figures . . . It can hardly be estimated how many of the 1359 (polio) cases among vaccinated persons must be regarded as failures of the vaccine and how many of them were infected by the vaccine. A careful study of the epidemiologic course of polio in the United States yields indications of grave significance. In numerous states of the U.S.A., typical early epidemics developed with the immunizations in the spring of 1955 . . . The vaccination incidents of the year 1955 cannot be exclusively traced back to the failure of one manufacturing firm."

Dr. Herbert Ratner, *Child and Family*, 1980, vol. 19, no. 4, "Story of the Salk Vaccine (Part 2)."

"Suffice it to say that most of the large (polio) epidemics that have occurred in this country since the introduction of the Salk vaccine have followed the wide-scale use of the vaccine and have been characterized by an uncommon early seasonal onset. To name a few, there is the Massachusetts epidemic of 1955; the Chicago epidemic of 1956; and the Des Moines epidemic of 1959."

Dr. Herbert Ratner, *Child and Family*, 1980 vol. 19, no. 4.

"The live (Sabin) poliovirus vaccine has been the predominant cause of domestically arising cases of paralytic poliomyelitis in the United States since 1972. To avoid the occurrence of such cases, it would be necessary to discontinue the routine use of live poliovirus vaccine."

Jonas Salk, *Science*, March 4, 1977, p. 845.

"By the (U.S.) government's own admission, there has been a 41% failure rate in persons who were previously vaccinated against the (measles) virus."[4]

Dr. Anthony Morris, John Chriss, BG Young, "Occurrence of Measles in Previously Vaccinated Individuals," 1979; presented at a meeting of the American Society for Microbiology at Fort Detrick, Maryland, April 27, 1979.

"Prior to the time doctors began giving rubella (measles) vaccinations, an estimated 85% of adults were naturally immune to the disease (for life). Because of immunization, the vast majority of women never acquire natural immunity (or lifetime protection)."

Dr. Robert Mendelsohn, *Let's Live*, December 1983, as quoted by Carolyn Reuben in the *LA Weekly*, June 28, 1985.

"Adminstration of KMV (killed measles vaccine) apparently set in motion an aberrant immunologic response that not only failed to protect children against natural measles, but resulted in heightened susceptibility."

JAMA Aug. 22, 1980, vol. 244, p. 804, Vincent Fulginiti and Ray Helfer. The authors indicate that such falsely protected children can

---

[4] The authors state they examined records for 26,795 cases of measles reported to the CDC circa 1978. Of these, they found that 7,230 had been previously vaccinated against measles. See *Public Scrutiny*, August 1979.

come down with "an often severe, atypical form of measles. Atypical measles is characterized by fever, headache . . . and a diverse rash (which) . . . may consist of a mixture of macules, papules, vesicles, and pustules . . . "

The above quotes reflect an available literature which shows there is a need for an extensive review of vaccination. It is certain that undisclosed, unlooked for illness occurs as a result of vaccines, or as a result of infection after protective immunity should have been but wasn't conferred.

A certain amount of this sort of illness is immunosuppressive in the widest sense, and some in a narrower sense (depression of T-cell numbers, etc.).

When looking for unusual illness and immune depression, vaccines are one of those areas which remain partially hidden from investigation. That is a mistake. Not enough is known about the effects of vaccines on the immune system. It is not adequate to say, "Vaccines are simple; they stimulate the immune system and confer immunity against specific agents."

That is the glossy presentation. What they apparently often do is something else. They engage some aspect of the body's immune-response, but to what effect over the long term? Why, for example, do children who have measles vaccine develop a susceptibility to another severe, atypical measles? Is that virulent form of the disease from within the result of reactivation of the virus in the old vaccine?

The following is a technical memorandum issued by the United States Congress' Office of Technology Assessment, dated November 1980. It is titled, "Compensation for Vaccine-Related Injuries," and contains a list of reported reactions to certain live vaccines (pages 42-43 are quoted in full). The left column indicates type of live vaccine.

	Known (reaction)	Probable (reaction)	Possible (reaction)
Measles	Fever	Encephalitis	Other Neurologic Disorders
	Rash	Encephalopathy	Guillain-Barre Syndrome
	Convulsions	Subacute Sclerosing	Transverse Myelitis
	(Primary Febrile)	Panencephalitis (SSPE)	Atixia
		Reye's Syndrome	Cranial Nerve Paralysis
			Teratogenesis
Mumps		Parotitis	Encephalitis, Aseptic
			Meningitis
			Unilateral Nerve Deafness
			Allergic Reactions
			Rash, Pruritis, Purpura
			Reye's Syndrome
			Deafness and Other
			Neurologic Disorder:
			-Teratogenesis
Rubella	Lymphadenopathy	Teratogenesis	Thrombocytopenia
	Fever		Encephalitis, Aseptic
	Rash		Meningitis
	Arthralgia		Other Neurologic
	Arthritis		Disorder
	Peripheral Nueitis		Transverse Myelitis
			Guillain-Barre
			Syndrome
			Hemiparesis
			Ataxia
			Convulsions
Polio	Paralytic Polio	Teratogenesis	Reye's Syndrome

	Known (reaction)	Probable (reaction)	Possible (reaction)
Smallpox	Local Infection (Pustule) Regional Lymphadenopathy Fever "Toxic" Eruption Dissemination and Eczema Vaccinatum	Encephalitis Encephalopathy	Transverse Myelitis Hemiplegia Reye's Syndrome Guillain-Barre Syndrome Teratogenesis
Diphtheria and Tetanus Toxoids and Pertussis Vaccine (DTP)	Local Swelling Sterile abscesses Fever Convulsions	Encephalopathy Encephalitis Persistent Screaming	Reye's Syndrome Guillain-Barre Syndrome Peripheral Neuritis
Tetanus Toxoid and Tetanus-Dephtheria Toxoids (T, DT, & Td) Adult	Hypersensitivity Local Reactions Fever Convulsions (Febrile)		Encephalitis, Aseptic Meningitis Other Neurologic Disorders Peripheral Neuropathy Cranial Nerve Palsy (Neuritis)
Polio Vaccine Inactivated (IPV)			Allergic Reactions Guillain-Barre Syndrome Teratogenesis (Neurogenic Tumors)
Influenza	Local Reactions Fever, Malaise Guillain-Barre Syndrome Allergic Reactions		Peripheral Neuropathy Neuritis

----

Official reports on vaccine reactions are often at odds with un-official estimates because of the method of analysis used. If vaccine-reaction is defined as a small set of possible effects experienced within 72 hours of an inoculation, then figures will be smaller. But doctors like G.T. Stewart, of the University of Glasgow, have found through meticulous investigation, including visits to hospitals and interviews with parents of children vaccinated, that reactions as severe as brain-damage (e.g., from the DPT vaccine) can be overlooked, go unreported and can be assumed mistakenly to have come from other causes. JR

APPENDIX 2

THE FIRST FIVE AIDS CASES

What follows is the first report of AIDS cases listed in a CDC Morbidity and Mortality Report (June 5, 1981). At the time of the report, these five men were not called AIDS patients. That came later.

Pneumocystis **Pneumonia–Los Angeles**

In the period October 1980-May 1981, 5 young men, all active homosexuals, were treated for biopsy-confirmed *Pneumocystis carinii* pneumonia at 3 different hospitals in Los Angeles, California. Two of the patients died. All 5 patients had laboratory-confirmed previous or current cytomegalovirus (CMV) infection and candidal mucosal infection. Case reports of these patients follow.

Patient 1: A previously healthy 33-year-old man developed *P. carinii* pneumonia and oral mucosal candidiasis in March 1981 after a 2-month history of fever associated with elevated liver enzymes, leukopenia, and CMV viruria. The serum complement-fixation CMV titer in October 1980 was 256; in May 1981 it was 32.[1] The patient's condition deteriorated despite courses of treatment with trimethoprim-sulfamethoxazole (TMP/SMX), pentamidine, and acyclovir. He died May 3, and postmortem examination showed residual *P. carinii* and CMV pneumonia, but no evidence of neoplasia.

Patient 2: A previously healthy 30-year-old man developed *P. carinii* pneumonia in April 1981 after a 5-month history of fever each day and of elevated liver-function tests, CMV viruria, and documented seroconversion to CMV, i.e., an acute-phase titer of 16 and a

---

[1] Paired specimens not run in parallel.

convalescent-phase titer of 28[2] in anticomplement immunofluorescence tests. Other features of his illness included leukopenia and mucosal candidiasis. His pneumonia responded to a course of intravenous TMP/SMX, but, as of the latest reports, he continues to have a
fever each day.

Patient 3: A 30-year-old man was well until January 1981 when
he developed esophageal and oral candidiasis that responded to Amphotericin B treatment. He was hospitalized in February 1981 for *P.
carinii* pneumonia that responded to oral TMP/SMX. His esophageal
candidiasis recurred after the pneumonia was diagnosed, and he was
again given Amphotericin B. The CMV complement-fixation titer in
March 1981 was 8. Material from an esophageal biopsy was positive
for CMV.

Patient 4: A 29-year-old man developed *P. carinii* pneumonia
in February 1981. He had had Hodgkins disease 3 years earlier, but
had been successfully treated with radiation therapy alone. He did
not improve after being given intravenous TMP/SMX and corticosteroids and died in March. Postmortem examination showed no evidence of Hodgkins disease, but *P. carinii* and CMV were found in
lung tissue.

Patient 5: A previously healthy 36-year-old man with a clinically diagnosed CMV infection in September 1980 was seen in April
1981 because of a 4-month history of fever, dyspnea, and cough. On
admission he was found to have *P. carinii* pneumonia, oral candidiasis, and CMV retinitis. A complement-fixation CMV titer in April
1981 was 128. The patient has been treated with 2 short courses of
TMP/SMX that have been limited because of a sulfa-induced neu-
tropenia. He is being treated for candidiasis with topical nystatin.

The diagnosis of *Pneumocystis* pneumonia was confirmed for
all 5 patients antemortem by closed or open lung biopsy. The patients
did not know each other and had no known common contacts or
knowledge of sexual partners who had had similar illnesses. The 5
did not have comparable histories of sexually transmitted disease.
Four had serologic evidence of past hepatitis B infection but had no

---

2 Ibid.

evidence of current hepatitis B surface antigen. Two of the 5 reported having frequent homosexual contacts with various partners. All 5 reported using inhalant drugs, and 1 reported parenteral drug abuse. Three patients had profoundly depressed numbers of thymus-dependent lymphocyte cells and profoundly depressed *in vitro* proliferative responses to mitogens and antigens. Lymphocyte studies were not performed on the other 2 patients.

Reported by MS Gottlieb, MD, HM Schanker, MD, PT Fan, MD, A Saxon, MD, JD Weisman, DO, Div of Clinical Immunology-Allergy, Dept of Medicine, UCLA School of Medicine; I Pozalski, MD, Cedars-Mt. Sinai Hospital, Los Angeles; Field Services Div, Epidemiology Program Office, CDC.

Editorial Note: *Pneumocystis* pneumonia in the United states is almost exclusively limited to severely immunosuppressed patients (1). The occurrence of pneumocystosis in these 5 previously healthy individuals without a clinically apparent underlying immunodeficiency is unusual. The fact that these patients were all homosexuals suggests an association between some aspect of a homosexual lifestyle or disease acquired through sexual contact and *Pneumocystis* pneumonia in this population. All 5 patients described in this report had laboratory-confirmed CMV disease or virus shedding within 5 months of the diagnosis of *Pneumocystis* pneumonia. CMV infection has been shown to induce transient abnormalities of *in vitro* cellular-immune function in an otherwise healthy human host (2, 3). Although all 3 patients tested had abnormal cellular-immune function, no definitive conclusion regarding the role of CMV infection in these 5 cases can be reached because of the lack of published data on cellular-immune function in healthy homosexual males with and without CMV antibody. In 1 report, 7 (3.6%) of 194 patients with pneumocystosis also had CMV infection; 40 (21%) of the same group had at least 1 other major concurrent infection (1). A high prevalence of CMV infections among homosexual males was recently reported: 179 (94%) of 190 males reported to be exclusively homosexual had serum antibody to CMV, and 14 (7.4%) had CMV viruria; rates for 101 controls of similar age who were reported to be exclusively heterosexual were 54% for seropositivity and zero for viruria (4). In another study of 64 males, 4 (6.3%) had positive tests for CMV in semen, but none had CMV recovered from urine. Two of the 4 reported recent homosexual contacts. These findings suggest not only that virus shedding may be more readily detected in seminal fluid than in urine, but also that seminal fluid may be an important vehicle of CMV transmission (5).

All the above observations suggest the possibility of a cellular-immune dysfunction related to a common exposure that predisposes individuals to opportunistic infections such as pneumocystosis and candidiasis. Although the role of CMV infection in the pathogenesis of pneumocystosis remains unknown, the possibility of *P. carinii* infection must be carefully considered in differential diagnosis for previously healthy homosexual males with dyspnea and pneumonia.

References

1. **Walzer PD, Perl DP, Krogstad DJ, Rawson PG, Schultz MG.** *Pneumocystis carinii* pneumonia in the United States. Epidemiologic, diagnostic, and clinical features. Ann Intern Med 1974; 80:83-93.

2. **Rinaldo CR, Jr, Black PH, Hirsch MS.** Interaction of cytomegalovirus with leukocytes from patients with mononucleosis due to cytomegalovirus. J Infect Dis 1977; 136:667-78.

3. **Rinaldo CR, Jr, Carney WP, Richter BS, Black PH, Hirsch MS.** Mechanisms of immunosuppression in cytomegaloviral mononucleosis. J Infect Dis 1980; 141:488-95.

4. **Drew WL, Mintz L, Miner RC, Sands M, Ketterer B.** Prevalence of cytomegalovirus infection in homosexual men. J Infect Dis 1981; 143:188-92.

5. **Lang DJ, Kummer JF.** Cytomegalovirus in semen: observations in selected populations. J Infect Dis 1975, 132:472-3.

My comment:

In the August 28, 1981, *Morbidity and Mortality Report*, two months after the above report, the CDC noted that more cases of pneumocystis, and also Kaposi's sarcoma, had been diagnosed in the U.S. All of these 26 cases, which included the first five, were, it said, "among previously healthy homosexual men . . ." That was incorrect.

In a following paragraph, we find this statement: "The occurrence of Pneumocystis carinii pneumonia among patients who are not immuno-suppressed due to known underlying disease or therapy is also highly unusual."

That is deceptive and incomplete. Pneumocystis has been found, for example, in children who are suffering from severe malnutrition. A correct statement would have been: Pneumocystis can apparently occur in patients who are severely immunosuppressed *for any reason*.

But at this point, the die was cast. Federal health agencies began to look for an underlying disease that gave rise to the pneumocystis. They assumed it existed and was the same in all cases. They would ultimately reject the idea that various chemicals and illnesses (STDs) in concert could cause pneumocystis to develop. They would opt for a solution that posited one novel universal agent, HIV. That decision may turn out to be the biggest mistake in the history of medicine.

As to the five homosexual men who, during the period October 1980-May 1981, were all admitted to Los Angeles hospitals and treated for pneumocystis, the CDC summary implies there was some history of sexually transmitted diseases among them. Sexually transmitted diseases (STDs), especially when combined with large amounts of antibiotics, can rank as immuno-suppressive, and it is common to find in AIDS patients extensive histories of STDs.

All of the Los Angeles patients reported histories of inhalant drugs, frequently used in the gay community.

Patient number one had leukopenia (impaired production of white blood cells), an immune disorder which can be caused by drugs for gonorrhea or gout. Whether these drugs had been prescribed in the past for this patient is not mentioned. The patient while in the hospital was given a course of treatment which included TMP/SMX, pentamidine and acyclovir. TMP/SMX causes, in some patients, drug fever, nerve and bone-marrow reactions, in which case the drug must be stopped. Pentamidine, in traditional doses, increases liver and kidney toxicity in about 25% of patients taking it. Acyclovir is given for herpes. It has, on rare occasion, caused cerebral endema, seizures and death.

Patient number one had also had, prior to hospital admission, "a 2-month history of fever associated with elevated liver enzymes," states the June 1981 CDC *Morbidity and Mortality Report*. This could mean hepatitis, heroin, alcoholism, and in any event, the lengthy fever certainly would have had a deleterious effect on his immune system. Apparently, no attempt was made to discover the cause of that fever, other than to propose a new virus.

Patient two had had a five-month history of fever prior to developing pneumocystis. That is a remarkably long time for a fever, and certainly signals an exhausted immune system. He also had elevated liver enzymes. Was he an alcoholic? The CDC report gives us no indication. This patient, as well as all of the others, had a previous (or current) case of CMV infection. Cytomegalovirus can cause pneumonia and blindness, among other symptoms, and several researchers are now beginning to wonder whether it has as much right to be called the cause of AIDS as HIV.

Patient two was also suffering from leukopenia. This patient received a course of TMP/SMX.

Patients three, four and five, aside from their inhalant drug use and CMV infection history, received such toxic treatments as corticosteroids (lowers the number of B and T immune-cells in the blood), radiation (for a past Hodgkins disease), and TMP/SMX (to which patient five had a severe reaction).

Amazingly, all of these patients were referred to by the CDC as "previously healthy." I now believe this is a technical term which means "not previously dead."

The implications were clear. Assumption number one: No multiple-cause scenarios explaining the pneumocystis and other infections would be accepted.

Assumption 2: The underlying cause of the Kaposi's sarcoma and pneumocystis (two very different diseases) would be taken to be the same in every case.

Assumption 3: The underlying cause would be a microbe.

Assumption 4: That microbe becomes (as of 1984, three years later) HIV.

In fact, and this is borne out in more vivid detail by later clinical evidence, many AIDS patients present vast amounts of varied *chemical* immune-suppression.

With all of the interviews and surveys that have been done of AIDS patients, outrageous histories of drug use have never been factored seriously into the equation as the prelude to the multiple-infection disaster called AIDS.

Nowhere is it clearer that such information is unwelcome than at the top of the research ladder, where Robert Gallo, number one U.S. AIDS researcher, works in his tumor lab at the National Cancer Institute. With a proprietary passion, Gallo protects "his" HIV virus from charges that it collaborates with factors in the lives and medical histories of some patients to produce disease. No cofactors, Gallo repeats. To have AIDS, you only need the virus.

Such unwarranted insistence contributes to the public fear that the virus can attack without notice and that AIDS is exactly nothing more than a randomly attacking infectious disease.

Seeing as he has never proved that HIV causes AIDS, or any disease, one can only wonder where Gallo's attitude is coming from – regarding the lack of need to investigate patient's backgrounds. Such investigation has been scotched, cut off at the top of the AIDS research ladder, where the biggest monies coagulate, where dictums are sent back down to the press, to the White House, universities and government health agencies.

APPENDIX 3

REVISION OF THE CDC
SURVEILLANCE CASE DEFINITION
FOR ACQUIRED IMMUNODEFICIENCY
SYNDROME (1987)

Introduction

The following revised case definition for surveillance of acquired immuno-deficiency syndrome (AIDS) was developed by CDC in collaboration with public health and clinical specialists. The Council of State and Territorial Epidemiologists (CSTE) has officially recommended adoption of the revised definition for national reporting of AIDS. The objectives of the revision are a) to track more effectively the severe disabling morbidity associated with infection with human immunodeficiency virus (HIV) (including HIV-1 and HIV-2); b) to simplify reporting of AIDS cases; c) to increase the sensitivity and specificity of the definition through greater diagnostic application of laboratory evidence for HIV infection: and d) to be consistent with current diagnostic practice, which in some cases includes presumptive, i.e., without confirmatory laboratory evidence, diagnosis of AIDS-indicative diseases (e.g., Pneumocystis carinii pneumonia, Kaposi's sarcoma).

The definition is organized into three sections that depend on the status of laboratory evidence of HIV infection (e.g., HIV antibody) (Figure). The major proposed changes apply to patients with laboratory evidence for HIV infection: a) inclusion of HIV encephalopathy, HIV wasting syndrome, and a broader range of specific AIDS-indicative diseases (Section II.A); b) inclusion of AIDS patients whose indicator diseases are diagnosed presumptively (Section II.B); and c) elimination of exclusions due to other causes of immunodeficiency (Section I.A).

309

Application of the definition for children differs from that for adults in two ways. First, multiple or recurrent serious bacterial infections and lymphoid interstitial pneumonia/pulmonary lymphoid hyperplasia are accepted as indicative of AIDS among children but not among adults. Second, for children less than 15 months of age whose mothers are thought to have had HIV infection during the child's perinatal period, the laboratory criteria for HIV infection are more stringent, since the presence of HIV antibody in the child is, by itself, insufficient evidence for HIV infection because of the persistence of passively acquired maternal antibodies less than 15 months after birth.

The new definition is effective immediately. State and local health departments are requested to apply the new definition henceforth to patients reported to them. The initiation of the actual reporting of cases that meet the new definition is targeted for September 1, 1987, when modified computer software and report forms should be in place to accommodate the changes. CSTE has recommended retrospective application of the revised definition to patients already reported to health departments. The new definition follows:

1987 REVISION OF CASE DEFINITION FOR AIDS FOR SURVEILLANCE PURPOSES

For national reporting, a case of AIDS is defined as an illness characterized by one or more of the following "indicator" diseases, depending on the status of laboratory evidence of HIV infection, as shown below.

I. Without Laboratory Evidence Regarding HIV Infection

If laboratory tests for HIV were not performed or gave inconclusive results (See Appendix I) and the patient had no other cause of immunodeficiency listed in Section I.A below, then any disease listed in Section I.B indicates AIDS if it was diagnosed by a definitive method (See Appendix II).

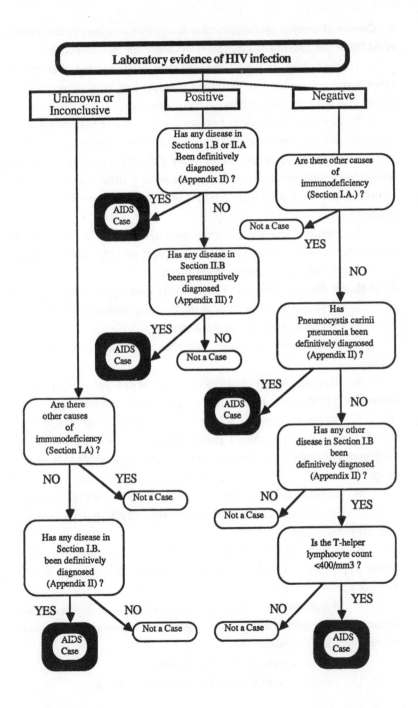

A. Causes of immunodeficiency that disqualify diseases as indicators of AIDS in the absence of laboratory evidence for HIV infection

    1. high-dose or long-term systemic corticosteroid therapy or other immunosuppressive/cytotoxic therapy less than or equal to 3 months before the onset of the indicator disease

    2. any of the following diseases diagnosed less than or equal to 3 months after diagnosis of the indicator disease: Hodgkin's disease, non-Hodgkin's lymphoma (other than primary brain lymphoma), lymphocytic leukemia, multiple myeloma, any other cancer of lymphoreticular or histiocytic tissue, or angioimmunoblastic lymphadenopathy

    3. a genetic (congenital) immunodeficiency syndrome or an acquired immunodeficiency syndrome atypical of HIV infection, such as one involving hypogammaglobulinemia

B. Indicator diseases diagnosed definitively (See Appendix II)

    1. Candidiasis of the esophagus, trachea, bronchi, or lungs

    2. Cryptococcosis, extrapulmonary

    3. Cryptosporidiosis with diarrhea persisting greater than 1 month

    4. Cytomegalovirus disease of an organ other than liver, spleen, or lymph nodes in a patient greater than 1 month of age

    5. Herpes simplex virus infection causing a mucocutaneous ulcer that persists longer than 1 month; or bronchitis, pneumonitis, or esophagitis for any duration affecting a patient greater than 1 month of age

    6. Kaposi's sarcoma affecting a patient less than 60 years of age

    7. Lymphoma of the brain (primary) affecting a patient less than 60 years of age

    8. Lymphoid interstitial pneumonia and/or pulmonary lymphoid hyperplasia (LIP/PLH complex) affecting a child less than 13 years of age

    9. Mycobacterium avium complex or M. kansasii disease, disseminated (at a site other than or in addition to lungs, skin, or cervical or hilar lymph nodes)

    10. Pneumocystis carinii pneumonia

    11. Progressive multifocal leukoencephalopathy

12. Toxoplasmosis of the brain affecting a patient greater than 1 month of age

II. With Laboratory Evidence for HIV infection

Regardless of the presence of other causes of immunodeficiency (I.A.), in the presence of laboratory evidence for HIV infection (See Appendix I), any disease listed above (I.B) or below (II.A or II.B) indicates a diagnosis of AIDS.

A. Indicator diseases diagnosed definitively (See Appendix II)

1. bacterial infections, multiple or recurrent (any combination of at least two within a 2-year period), of the following types affecting a child less than 13 years of age: septicemia, pneumonia, meningitis, bone or joint infection, or abscess of an internal organ or body cavity (excluding otitis media or superficial skin or mucosal abscesses), caused by Haemophilus, Streptococcus (including pneumococcus), or other pyogenic bacteria

2. coccidioidomycosis, disseminated (at a site other than or in addition to lungs or cervical or hilar lymph nodes)

3. HIV encephalopathy (also called "HIV dementia," "AIDS dementia," or "subacute encephalitis due to HIV") (See Appendix II for description)

4. histoplasmosis, disseminated (at a site other than or in addition to lungs or cervical or hilar lymph nodes)

5. isosporiasis with diarrhea persisting greater than 1 month

6. Kaposi's sarcoma at any age

7. lymphoma of the brain (primary) at any age

8. other non-Hodgkin's lymphoma of B-cell or unknown immunologic phenotype and the following histologic types: a. small noncleaved lymphoma (either Burkitt or non-Burkitt type) (See Appendix IV for equivalent terms and numeric codes used in the Internation Classification of Diseases, Ninth Revision, Clinical Modification) b. immunoblastic sarcoma (equivalent to any of the following, although not necessarily all in combination: immunoblastic lymphoma, large-cell lymphoma, diffuse histiocytic lymphoma, diffuse undifferentiated lymphoma, or high-grade lymphoma) (See Ap-

pendix IV for equivalent terms and numeric codes used in the International Classification of Diseases, Ninth Revision, Clinical Modification)

Note: Lymphomas are not included here if they are T-cell immunologic phenotype or their histologic type is not described or is described as "lymphocytic," "lymphoblastic," "small cleaved," or "plasmacytoid lymphocytic"

9. any mycobacterial disease caused by mycobacteria other than M. tuberculosis, disseminated (at a site other than or in addition to lungs, skin, or cervical or hilar lymph nodes)

10. disease caused by M. tuberculosis, extrapulmonary (involving at least one site outside the lungs, regardless of whether there is concurrent pulmonary involvement)

11. Salmonella (nontyphoid) septicemia, recurrent

12. HIV wasting syndrome (emaciation, "slim disease") (See Appendix II for description)

B. Indicator diseases diagnosed presumptively (by a method other than those in Appendix II)

Note: Given the seriousness of diseases indicative of AIDS, it is generally important to diagnose them definitively, especially when therapy that would be used may have serious side effects or when definitive diagnosis is needed for eligibility for antiretroviral therapy. Nonetheless, in some situations, a patient's condition will not permit the performance of definitive tests. In other situations, accepted clinical practice may be to diagnose presumptively based on the presence of characteristic clinical and laboratory abnormalities. Guidelines for presumptive diagnoses are suggested in Appendix III.

1. candidiasis of the esophagus

2. cytomegalovirus retinitis with loss of vision

3. Kaposi's sarcoma

4. lymphoid interstitial pneumonia and/or pulmonary lymphoid hyperplasia (LIP/PLH complex) affecting a child less than 13 years of age

5. mycobacterial disease (acid-fast bacilli with species not identified by culture), disseminated (involving at least one site other than or in addition to lungs, skin, or cervical or hilar lymph nodes)

6. Pneumocystis carinii pneumonia

7. toxoplasmosis of the brain affecting a patient greater than 1 month of age

III. With Laboratory Evidence Against HIV Infection

With laboratory test results negative for HIV infection (See Appendix I), a diagnosis of AIDS for surveillance purposes is ruled out unless:

A. all the other causes of immunodeficiency listed above in Section I.A are excluded; AND

B. the patient has had either:

1. Pneumocystis carinii pneumonia diagnosed by a definitive method (See Appendix II; OR

2. a. any of the other diseases indicative of AIDS listed above in Section I.B diagnosed by a definitive method (See Appendix II); AND

b. a T-helper/inducer (CD4) lymphocyte count less than 400/mm3.

Reported by Council of State and Territorial Epidemiologists; AIDS Program, Center for Infectious Diseases, CDC

COMMENTARY

The surveillance of severe disease associated with HIV infection remains an essential, though not the only, indicator of the course of the HIV epidemic. The number of AIDS cases and the relative distribution of cases by demographic, geographic, and behavioral risk variables are the oldest indices of the epidemic, which began in 1981 and for which data are available retrospectively back to 1978. The original surveillance case definition, based on then-available knowledge, provided useful epidemiologic data on severe HIV disease. To ensure a reasonable predictive value for underlying immunodeficiency caused by what was then an unknown agent, the indicators of

AIDS in the old case definition were restricted to particular opportunistic diseases diagnosed by reliable methods in patients without specific known causes of immunodeficiency. After HIV was discovered to be the cause of AIDS, however, and highly sensitive and specific HIV-antibody tests became available, the spectrum of manifestations of HIV infection became better defined, and classification systems for HIV infection were developed.2-5 It became apparent that some progressive, seriously disabling, and even fatal conditions (e.g., encephalopathy, wasting syndrome) affecting a substantial number of HIV-infected patients were not subject to epidemiologic surveillance, as they were not included in the AIDS case definition. For reporting purposes, the revision adds to the definition most of those severe non-infectious, non-cancerous HIV-associated conditions that are categorized in the CDC clinical classification systems for HIV infection among adults and children.4,5

Another limitation of the old definition was that AIDS-indicative diseases are diagnosed presumptively (i.e., without confirmation by methods required by the old definition) in 10%-15% of patients diagnosed with such diseases; thus, an appreciable proportion of AIDS cases were missed for reporting purposes.6,7 This proportion may be increasing, which would compromise the old case definition's usefulness as a tool for monitoring trends. The revised case definition permits the reporting of these clinically diagnosed cases as long as there is laboratory evidence of HIV infection.

The effectiveness of the revision will depend on how extensively HIV-antibody tests are used. Approximately one third of AIDS patients in the United States have been from New York City and San Francisco, where, since 1985, less than 7% have been reported with HIV-antibody test results, compared with greater than 60% in other areas. The impact of the revision on the reported numbers of AIDS cases will also depend on the proportion of AIDS patients in whom indicator diseases are diagnosed presumptively rather than definitively. The use of presumptive diagnostic criteria varies geographically, being more common in certain rural areas and in urban areas with many indigent AIDS patients.

To avoid confusion about what should be reported to health departments, the term "AIDS" should refer only to conditions meeting the surveillance definition. This definition is intended only to provide consistent statistical data for public health purposes. Clinicians will not rely on this definition alone to diagnose serious disease caused by HIV infection in individual patients because there may be additional information that would lead to a more accurate diagnosis. For example, patients who are not reportable under the definition because they have either a negative HIV-antibody test or, in the presence of HIV antibody, an opportunistic disease not listed in the definition as an indicator of AIDS nonetheless may be diagnosed as having serious HIV disease on consideration of other clinical or laboratory characteristics of HIV infection or a history of exposure to HIV.

Conversely, the AIDS surveillance definition may rarely misclassify other patients as having serious HIV disease if they have no HIV-antibody test but have an AIDS-indicative disease with a background incidence unrelated to HIV infection, such as cryptococcal meningitis.

The diagnostic criteria accepted by the AIDS surveillance case definition should not be interpreted as the standard of good medical practice. Presumptive diagnoses are accepted in the definition because not to count them would be to ignore substantial morbidity resulting from HIV infection. Likewise, the definition accepts a reactive screening test for HIV antibody without confirmation by a supplemental test because a repeatedly reactive screening test result, in combination with an indicator disease, is highly indicative of true HIV disease. For national surveillance purposes, the tiny proportion of possibly false-positive screening tests in persons with AIDS-indicative diseases is of little consequence. For the individual patient, however, a correct diagnosis is critically important. The use of supplemental tests is, therefore, strongly endorsed. An increase in the diagnostic use of HIV-antibody tests could improve both the quality of medical care and the function of the new case definition, as well as assist in providing counseling to prevent transmission of HIV.

References

1. World Health Organization. Acquired immunodeficiency syndrome (AIDS): WHO/CDC case definition for AIDS. WHO Wkly Epidemiol Rec 1986; 61: 69-72.

2. Haverkos HW, Gottlieb MS, Killen JY, Edelman R. Classification of HTLV-III/LAV-related diseases (Letter). J Infect Dis 1985; 152: 1095.

3. Redfield RR, Wright DC, Tramont EC. The Walter Reed staging classification of HTLV-III infection. N Engl J Med 1986; 314: 131-2.

4. CDC. Classification system for human T-lymphotropic virus type III/lymphadenopathy-associated virus infections. MMWR 1986; 35: 334-9.

5. CDC. Classification system for human immunodeficiency virus (HIV) infection in children under 13 years of age. MMWR 1987; 36: 225-30, 235.

6. Hardy AM, Starcher ET, Morgan WM, et al. Review of death certificates to assess completeness of AIDS case reporting. Pub Hlth Rep 1987; 102(4): 386-91.

7. Starcher ET, Biel JK, Rivera-Castano R, Day JM, Hopkins SG, Miller JW. The impact of presumptively diagnosed opportunistic infections and cancers on national reporting of AIDS (Abstract). Washington, DC: III International Conference on AIDS, June 1-5, 1987.

APPENDIX I
Laboratory Evidence For or Against HIV Infection

1. For Infection:

When a patient has disease consistent with AIDS:

a. a serum specimen from a patient greater than or equal to 15 months of age, or from a child less than 15 months of age whose mother is not thought to have had HIV infection during the child's perinatal period, that is repeatedly reactive for HIV antibody by a screening test (e.g., enzyme-linked immunosorbent assay (ELISA)), as long as subsequent HIV-antibody tests (e.g., Western blot, immunofluorescence assay), if done, are positive; OR

b. a serum specimen from a child less than 15 months of age, whose mother is thought to have had HIV infection during the child's perinatal period, that is repeatedly reactive for HIV antibody by a screening test (e.g., ELISA), plus increased serum immunoglobulin levels and at least one of the following abnormal immunologic test results: reduced absolute lymphocyte count, depressed CD4 (T-helper) lymphocyte count, or decreased CD4/CD8 (helper/suppressor) ratio, as long as subsequent antibody tests (e.g., Western blot, immunofluorescence assay), if done, are positive; OR

c. a positive test for HIV serum antigen; OR

d. a positive HIV culture confirmed by both reverse transcriptase detection and specific HIV-antigen test or in situ hybridization using a nucleic acid probe; OR

e. a positive result on any other highly specific test for HIV (e.g., nucleic acid probe of peripheral blood lymphocytes).

2. Against Infection:

A nonreactive screening test for serum antibody to HIV (e.g., ELISA) without a reactive or positive result on any other test for HIV infection (e.g., antibody antigen, culture), if done.

3. Inconclusive (Neither For nor Against Infection):

a. a repeatedly reactive screening test for serum antibody to HIV (e.g., ELISA) followed by a negative or inconclusive supplemental test (e.g., Western blot, immunofluorescence assay) without a positive HIV culture or serum antigen test, if done; OR

b. a serum specimen from a child less than 15 months of age, whose mother is thought to have had HIV infection during the child's perinatal period, that is repeatedly reactive for HIV antibody by a screening test, even if positive by a supplemental test, without additional evidence for immunodeficiency as described above (in 1.b) and without a positive HIV culture or serum antigen test, if done.

APPENDIX II
Definitive Diagnostic Methods for Diseases Indicative of AIDS

cryptosporidiosis
cytomegalovirus
isosporiasis
Kaposi's sarcoma
lymphoma
lymphoid pneumonia or hyperplasia
Pneumocystis carinii pneumonia
progressive multifocal leukoencephalopathy
toxoplasmosis

  microscopy (histology or cytology).

candidiasis

  gross inspection by endoscopy or autopsy or by microscopy (histology or cytology) on a specimen obtained directly from the tissues affected (including scrapings from the mucosal surface), not from a culture.

coccidioidomycosis
cryptococcosis
herpes simplex virus
histoplasmosis

  microscopy (histology or cytology), culture, or detection of antigen in a specimen obtained directly from the tissues affected or a fluid from those tissues.

tuberculosis
other mycobacteriosis
salmonellosis
other bacterial infection

  culture

HIV encephalopathy[1] (dementia)

  clinical findings of disabling cognitive and/or motor dysfunction interfering with occupation or activities of daily living, or loss of behavioral developmental milestones affecting a child, progressing over weeks to months, in the absence of a concurrent illness or condition other than HIV infection that could explain the findings.

---

[1] For HIV encephalopathy and HIV wasting syndrome, the methods of diagnosis described here are not truly definitive, but are sufficiently rigorous for surveillance purposes.

Methods to rule out such concurrent illnesses and conditions must include cerebrospinal fluid examination and either brain imaging (computed tomography or magnetic resonance) or autopsy.

HIV wasting syndrome[2]

findings of profound involuntary weight loss greater than 10% of baseline body weight plus either chronic diarrhea (at least two loose stools per day for greater than or equal to 30 days) or chronic weakness and documented fever (for greater than or equal to 30 days, intermittent or constant) in the absence of a concurrent illness or condition other than HIV infection that could explain the findings (e.g., cancer, tuberculosis, cryptosporidiosis, or other specific enteritis).

APPENDIX III
Suggested Guidelines for Presumptive Diagnosis of Diseases Indicative of AIDS

candidiasis of esophagus

a. recent onset of retrosternal pain on swallowing; AND

b. oral candidiasis diagnosed by the gross appearance of white patches or plaques on an erythematous base or by the microscopic appearance of fungal mycelial filaments in an uncultured specimen scraped from the oral mucosa.

cytomegalovirus retinitis

a characteristic appearance on serial ophthalmoscopic examinations (e.g., discrete patches of retinal whitening with distinct borders, spreading in a centrifugal manner, following blood vessels, progressing over several months, frequently associated with retinal vasculitis, hemorrhage, and necrosis). Resolution of active disease leaves retinal scarring and atrophy with retinal pigment epithelial mottling.

mycobacteriosis

microscopy of a specimen from stool or normally sterile body fluids or tissue from a site other than lungs, skin, or cervical or hilar lymph nodes, showing acid-fast bacilli of a species not identified by culture.

Kaposi's sarcoma

---

2 Ibid.

a characteristic gross appearance of an erythematous or violaceous plaque-like lesion on skin or mucous membrane. (Note: Presumptive diagnosis of Kaposi's sarcoma should not be made by clinicians who have seen few cases of it.)

lymphoid interstitial pneumonia

bilateral reticulonodular interstitial pulmonary infiltrates present on chest X ray for greater than or equal to 2 months with no pathogen identified and no response to antibiotic treatment.

Pneumocystis carinii pneumonia

a. a history of dyspnea on exertion or nonproductive cough of recent onset (within the past 3 months); AND

b. chest X-ray evidence of diffuse bilateral interstitial infiltrates or gallium scan evidence of diffuse bilateral pulmonary disease; AND

c. arterial blood gas analysis showing an arterial p02 of less than 70 mm Hg or a low respiratory diffusing capacity (less than 80% of predicted values) or an increase in the alveolar-arterial oxygen tension gradient; AND

d. no evidence of a bacterial pneumonia.

toxoplasmosis of the brain

a. recent onset of focal neurologic abnormality consistent with intracranial disease or a reduced level of consciousness; AND

b. brain imaging evidence of a lesion having a mass effect (on computed tomography or nuclear magnetic resonance) or the radiographic appearance of which is enhanced by injection of contrast medium; AND

c. serum antibody to toxoplasmosis or successful response to therapy for toxoplasmosis.

APPENDIX IV

Equivalent Terms and International Classification of Disease (ICD) Codes for AIDS-Indicative Lymphomas

The following terms and codes describe lymphomas indicative of AIDS in patients with antibody evidence for HIV infection (Section II.A.8 of the AIDS case definition). Many of these terms are obsolete or equivalent to one another.

ICD-9-CM (11978)

Codes:

200.0

Reticulosarcoma

lymphoma (malignant): histiocytic (diffuse) reticulum cell sarcoma: pleomorphic cell type or not otherwise specified

200.2

Burkitt's tumor or lymphoma

malignant lymphoma, Burkitt's type

ICD-O (Oncologic Histologic Types 1976)

Codes:

9600/3

Malignant lymphoma, undifferentiated cell type

non-Burkitt's or not otherwise specified

9601/3

Malignant lymphoma, stem cell type

stem cell lymphoma

9612/3

Malignant lymphoma, immunoblastic type

immunoblastic sarcoma, immunoblastic lymphoma, or immunoblastic lymphosarcoma

9632/3

Malignant lymphoma, centroblastic type

diffuse or not otherwise specified, or germinoblastic sarcoma: diffuse or not otherwise specified

9633/3

Malignant lymphoma, follicular center cell, non-cleaved

diffuse or not otherwise specified

9640/3

Reticulosarcoma, not otherwise specified

malignant lymphoma, histiocytic: diffuse or not otherwise specified reticulum cell sarcoma, not otherwise specified malignant lymphoma, reticulum cell type
9641/3
Reticulosarcoma, pleomorphic cell type
malignant lymphoma, histiocytic, pleomorphic cell type reticulum cell sarcoma, pleomorphic cell type
9750/3
Burkitt's lymphoma or Burkitt's tumor
malignant lymphoma, undifferentiated, Burkitt's type malignant lymphoma, lymphoblastic, Burkitt's type.

My comment:

I have re-printed the entire 1987 AIDS definition because many physicians have apparently not seen it, and because it is enlightening to realize how many diseases, infections, and therefore symptoms are being attributed to the underlying action of HIV.

APPENDIX 4

AMERICAN CORPORATIONS AND AIDS

In December, 1987, Allstate Insurance and *Fortune Magazine* sponsored a survey of top-executive personnel in 623 small, medium and large corporations.

The results were interesting. 2% of these businesses now give HIV tests to prospective employees, and 1% test current employees.

So on the one hand, there is a reluctance to move into testing. This is obviously linked to suits that could result – not the least of which would stem from false-positive results on the HIV blood tests.

An earlier Allstate Forum on AIDS in October of 1987 had issued this missive: "Testing to detect antibodies to HIV can show only the presence of antibodies. It will not show that the person is infected with or will contract AIDS ... As these tests (Elisa and Western blot) are applied to the general population without known risk behaviors for AIDS, the likelihood of false positive error increases greatly ... The initial reaction to a positive finding on an antibody test may lead to suicidal feelings or other extreme emotions."

Nevertheless, of the 623 corporations polled, there was evidence that top executives would like to use tests results, if a way could be found. If a test revealed a prospective employee was positive for HIV, 39% of those surveyed said their companies would reject that person. Only 23% said they would definitely hire the person.

Among companies in the South, 49% said they would reject an HIV-positive prospective employee. 55% of small corporations would reject such a person.

In addition, if by some means an HIV test were instituted, 61% of those polled felt the results should go both to the current employee tested and the employer. That figure jumped to 70% in Southern companies, and went to 78% in small corporations.

The gist was, if companies could get away with testing people, they wouldn't be eager to hire them if they were antibody-positive, and they would want to know the test results on anybody working for them.

It's probably accurate to infer that, were the government to install mandatory testing, or were states to implement versions of it among groups, corporations would back it, approve it, want it.

An article, "Panic Prevention," by Meryl Davids, in the March, 1987, *Public Relations Journal,* described a case of hysteria breaking out at a New England Telephone office when an employee with AIDS returned to work after winning a discrimination suit. Two-thirds of the office staff walked out, and returned only after the company put together a quick in-house seminar on AIDS backed up by people from Massachusetts General Hospital.

Davids follows this anecdote with the following: "As AIDS whirls across the country, a second epidemic – panic – is getting caught in its winds . . . Stricken employees returning to work are sometimes greeted by what amounts to a lynch mob."

The article states even employees *suspected* of having AIDS will find their fellow workers, in company after company, refusing to "work with or touch that person, or use the same bathroom, telephone, water fountain or pencil."

There is no list of companies given where hysteria has erupted, and only one or two anecdotes, but if the article is indicative of widespread employee attitudes, HIV testing and subsequent isolation or firing would be dearly desired – as long as someone *else* could mandate testing and do it and turn over the results to employers.

APPENDIX 5

THE HEPATITIS B VACCINE

The following is an unpublished article I wrote in September, 1987. As you'll see, it assumes that HIV is the AIDS virus, that HIV testing is reliable, and that AIDS is a distinct entity. Within these absurd facades, I develop the argument that attempts to prove hepatitis B vaccine is safe rest on incomplete, and sometimes careless science. It is a visible example of doubts put to rest by science based on partial proof only, which the scientific community accepts without question.

A decade ago, 1083 male homosexuals in good health were inoculated with an experimental vaccine against hepatitis B, an infectious viral disease. The trial was run at a prestigious research facility, the New York Blood Center.

From NY Blood Center accounts, results were very good: There was virtually full protection against hepatitis B, which reportedly was starting to run rampant through pockets of the U.S. gay community.

At that time, in 1978, AIDS was an uninvented word. And not until 1984 would HIV be isolated and labeled by Luc Montagnier and Robert Gallo. When AIDS crept into public view in 1979, and then gained wide attention in the early 80s, people began fearing the hepatitis B vaccine.

The reason? The vaccine had originally been made from blood of human donors, some of whom later turned out to be diagnosed with AIDS.

During the early 1980s, health workers, who were at risk for hepatitis B, were urged to take the new vaccine, but they stayed away from the product in droves. Dr. Robert Mendelsohn, Chicago medical heretic, points out that initially the U.S. Veteran's Administration expected to give 90,000 doses of the hepatitis B vaccine to its employees around the country. The response rate, though, by 1983, was only 30,000 doses. In the same year, 1200 University of Illinois health workers were pressured to take hepatitis B shots. Only 237 did.

In January, 1983, a year before the AIDS virus was discovered, Dr. John Finkbeiner, writing in *Medical World News,* warned that the hepatitis B vaccine "might be contaminated with a pathogen responsible for the acquired immune deficiency syndrome (AIDS) epidemic."

Dr. James Chin, head of Infectious Diseases for California's Dept. of Health Services, contacted the Centers for Disease Control (CDC) and asked for long-term tracking of hepatitis B vaccinees. His implication was quite clear: Maybe the vaccine was causing AIDS.

There were other factors that added to public worry. Alan Cantwell, a Los Angeles physician who authored the book, *AIDS, the Mystery and the Solution,* recalls that "the CDC, reporting on the first 26 cases of AIDS in the U.S., declared that 20 were from New York, and 6 were from San Francisco and Los Angeles. These were the three cities that carried out the most extensive early hepatitis B vaccine-trials. Then, all of the first 26 AIDS cases matched the profile of the volunteers in these same vaccine-trials: male, gay, under 40, well educated, and (mostly) white."

Dr. Cantwell adds: "AIDS was the first time doctors could recall working with a disease that seemed to be specific for a certain cultural group, *i.e.* male homosexuals." Good reason to look for a common environmental factor – for example, a contaminated vaccine.

In the meantime, throughout the early 1980s, researchers around the world were scrambling to make a connection between AIDS in Africa, which was overwhelmingly heterosexual, and AIDS in America. A sketchy scenario emerged: The AIDS microbe, jumping species from an African green monkey to an African human, eventually infected Haitians who were living in Central Africa, probably Zaire. The Haitians took AIDS home with them. It moved into their male bisexual community, where American homosexuals from New York and San Francisco picked it up. They had traveled to the "gay playground" of Haitian clubs on vacation.

There were variations on this plot. One, tentatively advanced by World Health Organization advisor, Jacques Leibowitch, had it that Cuban soldiers, hacking their way through the jungles of Angola in the 70s, brought the incubating AIDS microbe home with them. Eventually, some of these troops who were gay ended up on the Cuban-boatpeople crew that President Carter let into the U.S. AIDS spread from them into the American homosexual community.

These renditions of how AIDS moved had the effect of quelling fear that "American AIDS" was the product of the hepatitis B vaccine.

Still, to some, the idea of blaming an epidemic on the Cubans sounded like CIA disinformation. Then, of course, there was (and is) no proof that the AIDS germ actually came from a monkey in Africa. Many accounts in fact placed the world's first actual AIDS cases in the U.S.

Finally, a few epidemiologists asked the burning question, If AIDS came to Manhattan from Haiti, then why didn't it break out at the same time in New Orleans and Houston? Gay men from those cities were going to Haiti, too.

So there was good reason, among media monkey-speculations and quasi-scientific pronouncements on AIDS' origins, to wonder still about a possible tie between AIDS and the hepatitis B vaccine.

By the end of 1984, the newly discovered HIV virus was in the bag. Now researchers would really be able to check out this whole hepatitis vaccine business. Previously, the CDC had been issuing bland assurances that no harm was coming to the gay community, who were receiving very large numbers of hepatitis B inoculations. But now that the cause of AIDS was supposedly known, it would be a matter of one-two-three. Did the AIDS virus infect the hepatitis B vaccine? Was HIV passed on to vaccinees? Was there a large risk?

In 1984, Dr. Cladd Stevens, of the New York Blood Center, assembled 212 men out of the 1083 who had taken part in the original hepatitis B vaccine-trial. She searched through their progressive blood samples, which had been kept, since 1978, for followups – and she found that 85 of them, a hefty 40%, now had positive AIDS blood tests.

In a recent conversation, I asked Dr. Stevens how many of these men, up to the present, have been diagnosed with full-blown AIDS. She said, "We don't know. We're starting to find out now. We have to compare our code-names with those reported to the CDC over the years as AIDS cases. Those lists are confidentially held – but now I think we can finally use them for this purpose.[1]

So in 1987, we still don't know how many gay men from the NY hepatitis B vaccine-trial have been diagnosed with AIDS. This is a revelation. Convential wisdom has had it that only one or two of those volunteers have actually come to be labeled AIDS cases. In fact, in early 1987, several newspapers, including the *New York Times*, published reports that only one person from the NY hepatitis B vaccine trial had developed AIDS. This information was apparently based on an interview with Dr. Stevens. But in fact, the issue isn't open and shut. Not at all.

Back in February, 1985, two letters appeared in the *New England Journal of Medicine*. Many health professionals assumed they also closed the door on the potential connection between AIDS and the hepatitis B vaccine.

The first letter, written by Dr. Stevens and Robert Gallo, pointed out that, in the original hepatitis B vaccine-trial in New York, the men who were in the control group and received a placebo subsequently, over the next 4 years, tested positive for HIV at the same rate (40%) as those who had been given the vaccine. Therefore, the vaccine was as harmless as the placebo.

However, Dr. Stevens goes on to make a thoroughly disqualifying statement in her letter. She says that 30 of these placebo recipients "tended to have larger numbers of sex partners than those who were vaccinated." In other words, she is implying, they were more likely to test positive for HIV because of their lifestyle. This, in effect, was candidly admitting that the placebo-recipients were not a comparable group to the vaccine-recipients. The comparison was invalid; the whole study was skewed.

---

[1] As of February 1988, this still has not been done.

In the same issue of the *New England Journal,* Dr. Jules Dienstag wrote a letter defending the safety of the hepatitis B vaccine, too. He pointed to his own study of 200 health workers who had been given hepatitis B inoculations. After a year, *none* of them tested positive for the AIDS virus.

Dienstag was obviously suggesting that high-risk gay males from the original hepatitis B vaccine-trial had become infected with the AIDS virus because of their lifestyles, and not because of the vaccine. Meanwhile, his health workers, who did not engage in such high-risk behavior, remained "pure."

Dienstag's evidence is significant. But it by no means closed the door on the AIDS-hepatitis vaccine connection. Different batches of the same vaccine can and do have different contents. The batch given to the 1083 gay men in the NY trial could have been contaminated with AIDS, and the batch given to Dienstag's health workers could have been free from AIDS. Furthermore, there is no indication Dienstag asked his health workers if they were gay or heterosexual. If some were gay, this would raise the troubling issue of why gays *over there* became HIV antibody-positive and gays *over here* didn't. Maybe the batches of hepatitis B vaccine really were different.

Dr. Cantwell comments, "I know of no later *comprehensive* checking of the vaccine batches given to the volunteers in the early NY, San Francisco, and LA hepatitis B vaccine-trials. These batches, *all* of them that are still available, need to be examined by people who were not involved in the original trials, vaccine-research, or manufacture."

Experts have admitted that blood from donors who had the HIV virus was made into hepatitis B vaccine. So naturally a study has been put together to see whether HIV actually traveled into the hepatitis vaccine. The confident answer? No.

The problem was that apparently only two pools of vaccine-substance were checked over. Furthermore, people who did the checking had been involved in earlier vaccine-work on hepatitis B.

A key study, published in the *Journal of the American Medical Association,* on August 15, 1986, asserts that outside intruding AIDS viruses were and are inactivated during the three purification steps taken in production of hepatitis B vaccines.

However, in interviews with several virologists who have had experience in vaccine quality-control, the following emerged: Widely accepted protocol for inactivation of viruses isn't always reliable.

There was, for example, the famous Cutter Labs polio-vaccine case, well-documented, in which children contracted polio from Cutter's vaccinations. Yet in making the polio vaccine, Cutter had purified their product and inactivated poliovirus according to government regulations. But children turned out to be more sensitive than the government's requirements. Cutter paid out $3 million in damages.

Moreover, in attempting to inactivate foreign viruses like HIV, people who make vaccines sometimes err. They don't always follow protocol. The number of errors in this field should not be assumed to be trivial.

The HIV virus takes two forms in the human body. The so-called provirus form, according to several researchers, wouldn't be inactivated by standard vaccine-making protocol at all.

In other words, we could have a myth. The myth is one of assurance. It says, We know the hepatitis B vaccine is safe, it had nothing to do with AIDS. It says, There was a scare, an understandable one, but now that's all over. Everything is all right.

But is it? Dr. Mathilde Krim, one of the leading lights at the American Foundation for AIDS Research said to me: "In dealing with pharmaceutical interests . . . it's very hard to get into their stocks of (vaccines) and do an examination."

"You mean you'd need a Congressional edict?" I asked.

"That might not even do it," she said.

Money to protect, reputations to guard – these are, of course, basic economic and human givens. When, beyond that, there are gross errors and omissions in defending the safety of a medical product, you have to ask how much trouble there really is below the surface. Concerning the hepatitis B vaccine, I don't think we yet know.

A NOTE ON ALTERNATIVE THEORIES OF AIDS

Since it can't be said too many times, I'll say it again: There is no proof that AIDS is a single disease-entity or a syndrome caused by one agent.

Most alternative theories of how AIDS came to be assume that AIDS exists, it is one thing, the reports of cases around the world are accurate, and HIV-blood testing is accurate and meaningful. In other words, they take the existing myths about AIDS and plug in another virus or bacteria and say IT is the real cause of AIDS.

When you look at these various theories, they all have claims that they can explain the huge list of symptoms which are attributed to AIDS.

If we take a few of these "alternate germs," such as bovine leukemia, the syphilis spirochete, African Swine Fever, a microbe among housed monkeys called STLV-III, we find that, at first glance, they all seem to have caused some AIDS symptoms either inside or outside of labs.

Swine Fever has caused lymphadenopathy and wasting away among millions of pigs. In 1974, at the Yerkes Primate Center in Atlanta, bovine leukemia virus in milk killed two baby chimps, who contracted pneumocystis pneumonia. STLV-III may have helped cause, in primate-center monkeys, blood-immune disorders and a wasting away.

And a March, 1976, paper (*Arch Pathol Med.*, vol. 100, p. 163, Chandler et al) reveals that, in 1969, five years before the first chimp in the U.S. was thought to have died of pneumocystis, *four* chimps died of pneumocystis. One of these cases was a primate who had been experimentally inoculated 44 months before his death with *Treponema pallidum*, syphilis.

So the animal literature can be read several different ways. What else is new?

The point is, when you try to say that immune suppression, which gives rise to opportunistic infections, wasting away, pneumonia . . . when you say this immune suppression comes from one cause, one germ, you're asking for trouble. All over the world there is immune suppression, there is reduced T-cell function, reduced macrophage function, there is the sprouting of opportunistic infections. This is nothing new.

To define a syndrome so loosely that it virtually includes any sort of immune suppression ever seen – this is bound to fail. It just doesn't work.

Alternative theories, if they prove anything, make stronger the suggestion that AIDS is not one thing.

If it is not one thing, the use of the label is very misleading and harmful, particularly when it is said to represent an invariably fatal disease.

I've heard a researcher blandly say that cofactors like alcohol and heroin couldn't have anything to do with AIDS because people have been drinking and shooting for centuries. As if, because all the alcoholics *he* knows don't have multiple bacterial infections, none do. That's nonsense. Some people react to prolonged alcohol in exactly that way, and the old term "wasted junky" isn't just social slang. Not all junkies simply linger in a perfectly preserved, forever sealed state of nothing. Some waste away and die.

I've heard a doctor point out that AIDS immune suppression was "different" because, in contrast to leukemia cases who were chemotherapied to their eyeballs, had no immune systems left — and yet developed no opportunistic infections — AIDS patients had infections coming out of every organ in their bodies.

As a matter of fact, the increase in pneumocystis pneumonia in this country, which started in 1956, was in part due to children with leukemia who were getting chemotherapy at hospitals all over America. They were coming down with pneumocystis. Check the literature. Ask the doctors.

Nevertheless, several of these germs, particularly Swine Fever and Syphilis, should be tracked down carefully, to see how much damage they have been causing humans.

A LETTER TO THE *PEOPLE WITH AIDS COALITION,* WRITTEN BY MICHAEL CALLEN

Michael Callen's letter is reprinted with his kind permission. It appeared in a recent issue of *Newsline,* which is available by subscription from the PWA Coalition, 263 A West 19th Street, Room 125, New York, NY. 10011.

Callen writes:

I received *one* response to my December column, "Why I Do Not Believe HIV is the Cause of AIDS, and Why I Think It Matters." The writer expressed interest in knowing what I *do* think is causing AIDS.

It's complicated. One advantage of believing that HIV is the cause of AIDS is that it's such a simple explanation. All you have to say is that a killer virus is on the loose which, like some PAC MAN video game, eats T-4 cells. Such a simplistic explanation seems tailor made for the TV age since it fits so beautifully into the 8 second sound bit mentality of most Americans.

I am a multifactorialist. I believe that *multiple* factors conspire to produce the immune deficiency which we now call AIDS. What seems to shock most people is that I do not believe that the causes (*plural!*) of AIDS are necessarily the same for the different risk groups. The reasons why an urban gay man gets AIDS may not be the same as why an IV drug user or hemophiliac gets AIDS.

The differences between the expression of AIDS in the different risk groups have always struck me as more important than the similarities. The median age differs by risk group; members of other risk groups almost never get KS (which is confined almost exclusively to gay men). And of course, the survival rates seem very different for different risk groups. How come the rate of antibody positivity among hemophiliac users of Factor 8 is so high while the rate of actual progression to AIDS is dramatically lower than in other risk groups? And now that we have both HIV-1 and HIV-2, we're being asked to believe that two viruses whose genetic make-ups are different enough to consider them different viruses could appear at the same time and happen to cause the same disease.

The strongest evidence against the idea of a unique, single viral cause for AIDS always seemed to me to be the epidemiology: the pattern of spread, particularly in the first three years of the epidemic.

If AIDS were truly caused by one virus, we ought to have seen cases of AIDS appear *simultaneously* in every major city where there are gay men and IV drug users. If HIV causes AIDS, why didn't gay men from Cincinnati and Des Moines who had spent their week's vacation in the Mineshaft get AIDS in 1981 and '82? Why were the overwhelming majority of all cases of AIDS confined almost exclusively to New York, San Francisco and Los Angeles for the first several years of this epidemic? Given the travel patterns of gay men in the late '70s and early '80s, any disease with a single viral cause ought to have spread in a "sweepstakes dispersal" pattern, instead of being so rigidly confined to three cities. One might have expected *fewer* cases in Cincinnati in 1982, but not *no* cases.

The discovery of HIV antibodies in the stored samples of the St. Louis teenager who died in the '60s suggests that HIV has been around longer than had been expected. Those who propose HIV as "the cause" of AIDS must explain why the epidemic waited so long to appear.

What about AIDS in IV drug users? Before the champions of HIV took over so completely, multifactorialists suggested that IV drug users had probably been dying of what we now call AIDS for years. Arrogant doctors scoffed: they would have seen it and reported it. But recently, New York City's Department of Health made headlines by announcing that a review of autopsy records indicates that thousands of deaths among IV drug users may in fact be related to what we now call AIDS. Now that doctors are *looking* for PCP (pneumocystis carinii pneumonia) under every rock, they're shocked to find so much of it. It may well have always been there (though undoubtedly there's more of it today than before).

To oversimplify, I believe that what others glibly refer to as "cofactors" may actually be the causes of AIDS. The immunosuppressive environmental and lifestyle factors which some scientists say "predispose" risk groups to infection with HIV may *by themselves* be sufficient to produce what we now call AIDS. They can destroy the immune system *without* having to invoke another virus to explain the damage.

Opiates and other IV drugs have long been known to be immunosuppressive. Sharing needles introduces foreign blood into the system; this is similar to getting a tissue transplant. The body mounts an attack on the foreign tissue. The blood in a shared needle undoubtedly contains all the infectious pathogens likely to be found in an IV drug user's blood: cytomegalovirus (CMV), various strains of hepatitis, Epstein-Barr virus, herpes, various bacterias and funguses and heaven only knows what else.

In terms of gay men, the body responds to semen and seminal fluid deposited in the rectum much like a kidney transplant. The semen is recognized as foreign tissue and the body mounts an attack which is immunocompromising. The use of immunosuppressive recreational drugs in the late '70s reached extraordinary levels. A number of infectious diseases became epidemic among a subset of sexually active urban gay men, the most important of which were probably hepatitis and CMV. One can be multiply and repeatedly infected with CMV; and infection by CMV causes immunosuppression and reactivations of EBV (Epstein-Barr Virus).

As for transfusion recipients, one must first ask what illness or trauma led to the need for a transfusion in the first place. Blood transfusions have *always* been risky because blood is dirty. Long before AIDS, there was always some degree of mortality associated with receiving blood transfusions. What we now call AIDS in transfusion recipients may well be a new name given to an old problem.

The most articulate and earliest explanation of the multifactorial hypothesis was published in the Annals of the New York

Academy of Sciences, Vol 437 (1984), pp. 177-183 and co-authored by Dr. Joseph Sonnabend, Steven Witkin, Ph.D. and Dr. David Purtilo. See also **The Acquired Immune Deficiency Syndrome and Infections of Homosexual Men**, edited by Pearl Ma, MD and Donald Armstrong, MD, (1983) pp. 409-425. For an intriguing overview of various hypotheses, see **AIDS Research**, Vol. 1, (1984), pp. 107-120. So many of the predictions made in that report have come true.

Were the multifactorialists put out of business by Dr. Gallo and Secretary Heckler's flashy press conference hastily called to announce what turned out to be the...[disputed discovery] of LAV[1] from the French? Everyone needed to believe that American science would get us out of this mess. America wanted a simple answer. HIV fit the bill, even though there were gaping holes in the simplistic assertion that HIV, acting alone (as Dr. Gallo arrogantly asserted) could explain a disease as complicated as AIDS.

There are a number of ways to generate a new disease. Of course, the introduction of a new virus into a virgin population is one way. But another way is a new configuration of old elements. CMV has been around forever. Gay men have been fucking forever. But never have CMV and gay fucking been brought together to quite the same degree as they were due to the historically unprecedented promiscuity of the late '70s. Never before in history had so many men had so much sex with each other, thanks to the commercialization of sex offered by a well-developed circuit of bathhouses and backrooms which existed in precisely those cities where AIDS first exploded. The median number of lifetime sexual partners for the first cohort of gay men with AIDS studied by the CDC was a staggering 1,150. That's not just any gay man; that's a specific subset of us. I'm not saying there's anything *morally* wrong with being promiscuous. But it's a fact that the more different partners one has, the more one increases one's chances of contracting an STD. Having 100 sex partners in Des Moines will probably only net you a head cold. But having that same number in Manhattan in 1981, where so many diseases

---

[1] The French title for HIV.

had reached epidemic proportions, would undoubtedly have had much more serious health consequences.

Everybody likes to compare AIDS in America with AIDS in Africa. Here's the only link I see: A small subset of highly promiscuous, urban gay men unwittingly managed to recreate disease settings equivalent to those of poor third world nations and junkies. My own case is a good example. By the age of 27, I estimate that I had had 3,000 different sex partners. I'd also had: hepatitis A, hepatitis B, hepatitis non-A, non-B; herpes simplex types 1 and 2; shigella; entomoeba histolitica; giardhia; syphilis; gonorrhea; non-specific urethritis; chlymidia; venereal warts; CMV; EBV-reactivations; and finally cryptosporidiosis and AIDS. The question for me wasn't why I was sick with AIDS but rather how I had been able to remain standing on two feet for so long. If you blanked out my name and handed my medical chart prior to AIDS to a doctor, she/he might reasonably have guessed that it was the chart of a 65 year old equatorial African living in squalor! Have we forgotten how much time we spent in our doctors' offices.

The very term "promiscuity" was a loaded word, one which had been used by right wing homophobes to beat gay people over the head. The fact that we multifactorialists were ourselves gay didn't cut any ice. We were blasted as suffering from internalized homophobia and guilt. Although everyone objected to its use ("What do you *mean*?"), everyone seems to have understood *exactly* what we meant by "promiscuity."

The political implications of the multifactorial hypothesis were less palatable than the HIV hypothesis. If HIV is *the* cause of AIDS, AIDS might just as easily have dropped into the community of housewives in Des Moines; it just *happened* to drop into the gay community first. HIV and AIDS are something that happened *to* us; not something we bear any responsibility for.

I use the analogy of a smoker who smoked 2 packs a day who ends up with lung cancer at the age of 50. Like the smoker, I believe that promiscuous gay men must bear some responsibility for developing AIDS. But no one bursts into the *smoker's* hospital room and screams: You've gotten what you deserved; we're not going to treat you; no more money for cancer research because you've brought it on yourself. No, this is America where Congress supports the tobacco subsidies *and* increases funding for cancer research. But AIDS involves sex, not tobacco, so of course America's response is irrational.

Because AIDS first struck gay men, homophobes used the notion that promiscuous gay people brought AIDS on themselves to justify no money for AIDS research and no compassion for PWAs. In this right wing atmosphere, with Buckley seriously proposing that antibody statuses be tattooed on each individual, those of us who believed in multifactorial etiology were censored or castigated for daring to air our views in public.

Where the smoking analogy doesn't fit concerns the fact that there are health warnings on every pack of cigarettes. No gay man in the '70s could have *dreamed* that the consequences of all those sexually transmitted diseases and drug use might be something as horrible as AIDS. Even if we multifactorialists prove to be right, issues of guilt and blame are *wholly* inappropriate. But acknowledging some responsibility is a different matter. And responsibility implies that one can *do* something to change the situation, such as safer sex.

Here, the multifactorial model posed an obvious advantage. If AIDS was the result of *repeated* exposures to immunosuppressive influences, then no single sexual encounter could give one AIDS. By contrast, I have never understood how those who have proposed that a *single* unlucky contact with HIV can lead to AIDS and death can recommend safer sex. I for one don't believe sex is worth dying for. If I thought a single sexual encounter could kill, I'd advise everyone to stop absolutely and completely until we have a cure or a vaccine. If sex is truly Russian Roulette as the proponents of HIV imply, then the only ethical advice would be to throw the gun away – not merely play less often. I know it offends some, but I think AIDS is a pretty hard disease to contract; you almost have to *work* at it to get it. This is strong evidence in favor of the multifactorial model.

Trying to convince America that everyone is equally at risk for AIDS has been a successful fundraising ploy. But it has also caused a lot of panic and needless social disruption. Many people who are the unlikeliest candidates to ever develop AIDS are nevertheless suffering tremendously from the fear of AIDS. Houses get burned down that way.

The truth has an odd way of rising to the surface. Whatever is *truly* causing AIDS will continue to cause AIDS regardless of what a majority of researchers prefer to *believe* is causing AIDS. The heretofore impenetrable edifice of HIV is crumbling before our eyes. Not just because Professor Duesberg of UC Berkeley has published a devastating refutation of HIV in a respected medical journal. Researchers have long been privately questioning certain HIV-related assumptions. And the much vaunted heterosexual AIDS explosion, transmission from women to men, is just not materializing. And one can only stretch that embarrassingly elastic "incubation period" so far before it snaps.

I admit that a virus called HIV is definitely present in the blood of a lot of people. But not in all people with AIDS. Not all people with HIV get sick. I admit that there's circumstantial evidence implicating HIV. But correlation is not causation.

I've been sick for 5 1/2 years now. I don't want to die. My life is worthy of the best science conducted by the classic rules of scientific inquiry. The deafening silence in response to Professor Duesberg's devastating challenge to HIV is a scandal! Science doesn't progress by ignoring embarrassing criticisms of received wisdom. If Duesberg is wrong, his claims should be easy to refute. Duesberg's devastating challenge to HIV has gone unanswered long enough. Join me in demanding that the authorities explain why Duesberg is wrong. If we multifactorials are right, the stakes are too high to keep pretending that we know what causes AIDS.

Since Callen's above letter was published in *Newsline*, Duesberg has testified before the Presidential Commission on AIDS. He was met with simplistic criticisms, and was given no chance to answer. There wasn't the slightest intimation that truth was the object of the exercise. JR

About The Author

Jon Rappoport is an investigative reporter. His articles on politics, environmental issues, and the arts have appeared in the *LA Weekly*, *Stern*, *In These Times*, *College Woman* and many other magazines and newspapers in the US and Europe. He lives in Los Angeles.

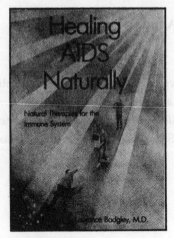

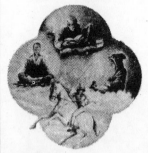